NATURAL CURES

DISCOVER THE POWERS OF FRUITS AND VEGETABLES

HEALTHY FOODS - HEALTHY EATING NOW!

NATURAL FOODS TO FEEL BETTER NOW

Your Natural Cures Superfoods

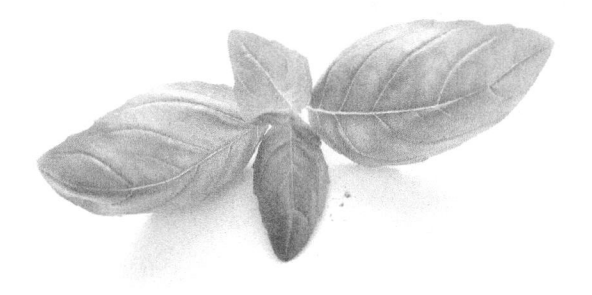

Copyright, Legal Notice and Disclaimer:

This publication is protected under the US Copyright Act of 1976 and all other applicable international, federal, state and local laws, and all rights are reserved, including resale rights: you are not allowed to give or sell this Guide to anyone else.

Please note that much of this publication is based on research, personal experience and anecdotal evidence. Although the author and publisher have made every reasonable attempt to achieve complete accuracy of the content in this Guide, they assume no responsibility for errors or omissions. Also, you should use this information as you see fit, and at your own risk. Your particular situation may not be exactly suited to the examples illustrated here; in fact, it's likely that they won't be the same, and you should adjust your use of the information and recommendations accordingly.

Any trademarks, service marks, product names or named features are assumed to be the property of their respective owners, and are used only for reference. There is no implied endorsement if we use one of these terms.

Finally, use your head. Nothing in this Guide is intended to replace common sense, legal, medical or other professional advice, and is meant to inform and entertain the reader. So have fun with this complete NATURAL CURES guide.

Copyright © 2014 Mario Fortunato. All rights reserved worldwide.

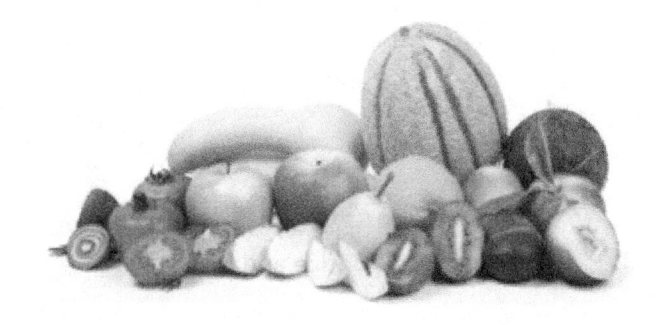

Table of Content:

- Introduction
- 11 Reasons of Why You Should Choose Fruits and Vegetables
- Discover the Powers of Purple Cabbage
- Discover the Powers of Zucchini
- Discover the Powers of Apples
- Discover the Powers of Oranges
- Discover the Powers of Peaches
- Discover the Powers of Pears
- Discover the Powers of Blackberries
- Discover the Powers of Strawberries
- Discover the Powers of Grapes
- Discover the Powers of Cherries
- Discover the Powers of Water Melon
- Discover the Powers of Bananas
- Discover the Powers of Mangosteen
- Discover the Powers of Mandarins
- Discover the Powers of Lemons
- Discover the Powers of Papaya
- Discover the Powers of Pineapples
- Discover the Powers of Mangoes
- Discover the Powers of Avocados

- [Discover the Powers of Pomegranate](#)
- [Discover the Powers of Onions](#)
- [Discover the Powers of Carrots](#)
- [Discover the Powers of Broccoli](#)
- [Discover the Powers of Spinach](#)
- [Discover the Powers of Santol](#)
- [Discover the Powers of Tomatoes](#)
- [Discover the Powers of Maca](#)
- [Discover the Powers of Garlic](#)
- [Discover the Powers of Ginger](#)
- [Discover the Powers of Kiwi](#)
- [List of the Amount of Fiber Contained in Fruits & Vegetables](#)
- [What are Antioxidants and Why We Need Them?](#)

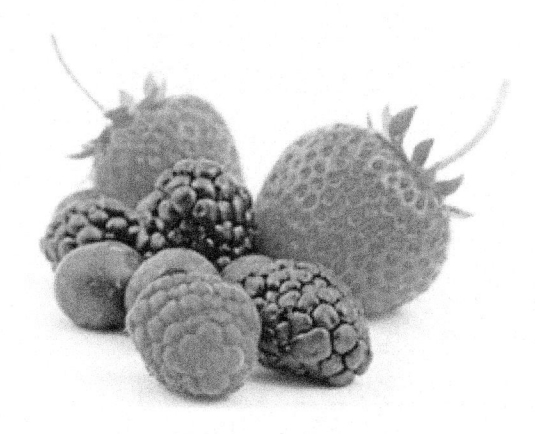

Introduction:

We definitively know that not all the answers for treating diseases and to achieve a healthier body can be found with traditional medicine. Oftentimes the use of chemicals and drug based treatments only worsen health problems when the real answer can be found in nature by **consuming lots of fresh fruits and vegetables**. Fruits and vegetables are full of nutrients and powerful antioxidants that will cure and prevent many diseases like cancer.

The secret of eating fruits and vegetables to improve your overall health is not just filling your body with these natural foods. One of the best and most effective secrets to get all the benefits from fruits and vegetables is to **eat them on an empty stomach**. By doing this your will get most of the health powers that these delicious and healthy foods can provide to our bodies. Nothing is easier to process or to digest for our human body than a fruit or a vegetable. Also the best way to consume these magical and healthy superfoods is by eating them in their raw state to profit from all the nutrients and the powers they have, when cooked some of the nutrients and vitamins are lost.

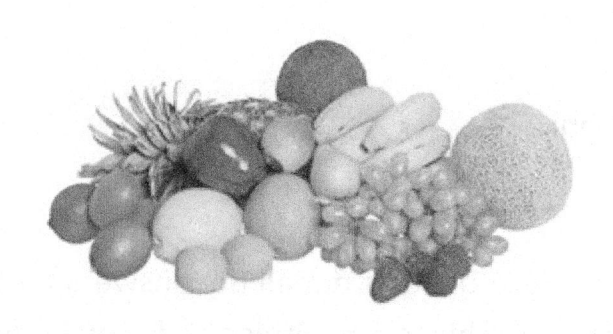

Always drink plenty of pure water with your fruits and vegetables to make your digestive system to work even better. **There is no better way to maintain a healthy body than by eating these powerful healthy foods.** There are plenty of good reasons to include fruits and vegetables in your daily diet. **Fruits and vegetables contain lots of dietary fiber**; this is excellent to keep a slim and energetic body. The fiber inside fruits makes you feel full and you lose weight faster. Fruits contain natural sugars that boost your energy levels naturally and effectively. **Fruits and vegetables are the best source of vitamins and nutrients** you can find in nature to keep a healthy, stronger and younger body. You reduce the risk of many types of diseases like different types of cancer and heart disease when you make these wonderful nourishments a part of your daily menus. **Stay healthy and stay younger** with the revealed powers of the best fruits and vegetables you will find in this book. You are responsible for your health and your health is the biggest asset you must to take care of today! Protect your health and keep doctors away!

We must increase the amount of fresh fruits and vegetables we eat if we want to stay healthy. These powerful superfoods should be the foundation of a healthier you and a healthy diet. **Phytochemicals** inside fruits and vegetables **help to fight tons of illnesses** like different types of cancers, high blood pressure, high cholesterol levels, diabetes and others. Phytochemicals are the substances that give fruits and vegetables their beautiful colors and powerful properties. Low in calories, **high in nutrients, vitamins and fiber**, there is no better type of food you can find in the entire nature than fruits and vegetables **discover all their powers** in this practical book that will reveal all the benefits you can get when you make them a part of your life. Fruits and vegetables are the best choice for an **anti-cancer diet**, to lower cholesterol naturally and to live longer and healthier.

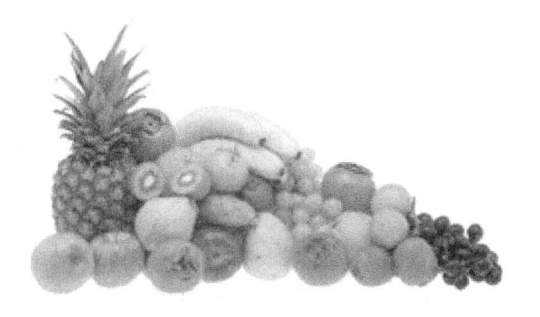

Eating healthier is being healthy and eating healthy means including at least 5 to 9 portions of different fresh fruits and vegetables every day. You can have a combination of different fruits or vegetables in the form of natural juices, in their raw state or prepared with salads. People who include these healthy superfoods in their diets tend to **live longer lives** and they have more energy. One way to ensure that you increase the consumption of these nourishments is by adopting the healthy habit of supplement all your meals with them. Instead of unhealthy sodas prefer fruit juices without any added sugar. Always **take them as a healthy snack** whenever you can and inspire kids to eat them too so they can replace candies with a healthier choice and get used to eating what is good for them.

The sad reality is that today most people don´t include these powerful superfoods into their diets and this is why people are getting sick because of the lack of good nutrients in their menus. People make all sorts of excuses of why they are not eating enough fruits and vegetables but the truth is that it is a matter of culture to get used to consume these healthy foods. Once you start to introduce these superfoods more and more into your daily menus

you will start to see your health positively changed forever literally. In fact different studies have shown that people over the age of 50 that start to consume more of these natural nourishments can significantly reduce the risk to develop different types of cancers and other diseases. So there is no excuse for not including **the best and most powerful type of delicious foods** you can find in nature in your daily diet, you can always come up with great new ideas on how to eat them each and every day.

Those who eat them are going to be blessed with all the benefits they have to offer and those who avoid them are going to regret it, there is no other healthier food choice in nature than fruits and vegetables, period.

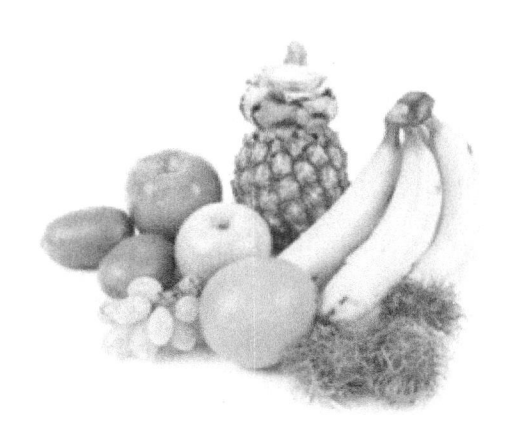

According to some recent studies the majority of people in the US and in other parts of the world are eating less than the recommended amount of fruits and vegetables to maintain a healthy body. **On a 2000 calories daily diet at least 2½ cups should be vegetables and at least 2 cups of fruits.** One way to ensure you consume this amount of these powerful healthy foods is to calculate that half of your plate should be filled with them in every meal you take during the day.

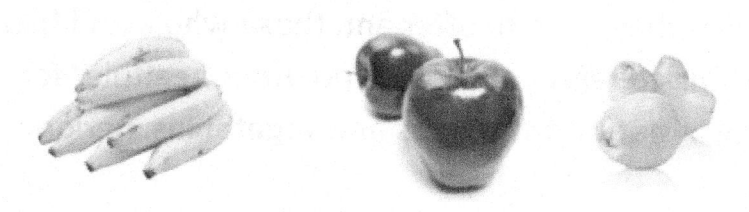

11 Reasons of Why You Should Choose Fruits and Vegetables

1. Fruits are full of flavor and color: they are a wonderful mosaic of various vivid colors that also have a natural sweet delicious taste as they contain natural sugars such as fructose, glucose and sucrose.
2. They can be consumed at any time of day; they are a

marvelous natural snack you can eat without worries of harming the health of your body and without the fear of getting obese. It's the best healthy snack you can eat that can bring your our body tons of essential vitamins and minerals.

3. They are a wonderful source of antioxidants: natural compounds contained inside these superfoods transform them into powerful antioxidants that slow cellular aging and protect the body from many degenerative diseases such as cancer.

4. These foods are rich in vitamins: both vegetables and fruits are full of vitamins that no other food can supplement in the same proportions. Always include some fruit or veggie in your daily menu that supplies your body with vitamin C to boost your immune system naturally. Inside this group are citrus fruits such as oranges, tangerines, grapefruit, lemon, kiwi, cantaloupe, strawberries, guava and pineapple.

5. Provides total hydration your body: the high content of H2O of fruits and vegetables facilitates the elimination of toxins from the body and help keep us well hydrated throughout the day.

6. They are a very flexible kind of natural food: you can mix them in many diverse ways with other foods to spice up numerous healthy recipes; you just have to let your imagination fly. However it is better to consume these superfoods in their raw state to retain all their antioxidant, detoxifying and healing powers. Although these foods can also be used in some healthy recipes that are cooked and they maintain their nutritional properties.

7. Both fruit and vegetables can be eaten at any time of the year and they are always available no matter season of year we are in, you can always choose seasonal fruits or those you love most.

8. These superfoods are naturally low-fat: it is almost imperceptible the amount of fat they have. The only ones with a high-fat are avocados and olives but these are healthy fruits and vegetables containing oleic acid fat.

9. They are good for removing excess fluids from the body and to prevent fluid retention: these superfoods contain very little sodium and potassium, this causes the body to eliminate fluids naturally and effectively.

10. They are rich in fiber that helps regulate bowel function, to cure constipation and to prevent obesity and diabetes. So eat as many fruits and vegetables as you can, your body and your health will thank you forever!

11. Another powerful reason for eating these superfoods is that they come in their own natural packaging and do not pollute the planet!

The **ideal consumption** fruits and vegetables a day **should be about five servings** and this equates to about 600 to 1000 grams per day of these foods. One serving of vegetables equals 150 to 200 grams which is equal to a bowl of mixed salad with a tomato, an eggplant, two cucumbers or 2 carrots.

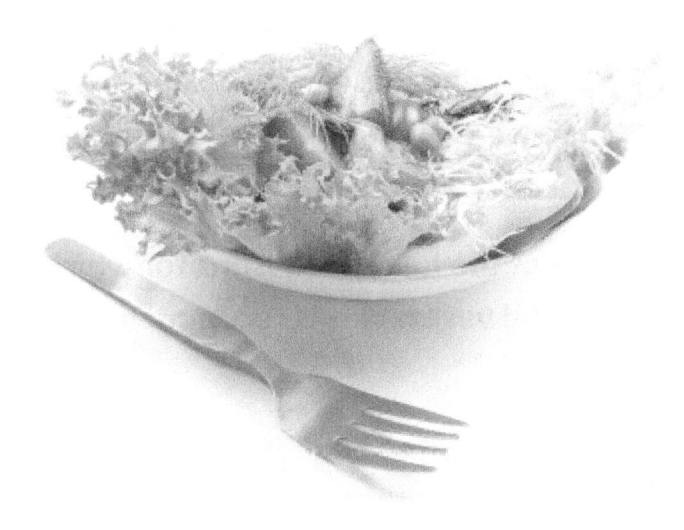

One serving of fruit can be composed of a pear, an orange, an apple and a banana or a grapefruit. **Why consume five servings?** Because they provide to our bodies important vitamins and minerals and are rich in antioxidants like vitamin C, folic acid and many other vitamins that improve our overall health. They also have fat-soluble vitamins like **carotenoids (beta-carotene)** and vitamin K vitamin A and E, and minerals such as potassium, magnesium and small amounts of calcium, phosphorus and iron. They contain **phytochemicals** that are organic compounds of vegetal origin that exert beneficial effects on human health. Fresh fruits can be consumed in their natural state or in the form of healthy natural juices, or crushed or mixed with healthy salads. Fresh vegetables can be eaten in salads, inside healthy soups, baked, boiled or steamed. You can use a vegetable steamer for cooking these natural superfoods and preserve their nutritional value.

This are some of the healthy reasons for which eating fruits and vegetables is recommended:

Our entire body gets the benefits when we eat these super healthy foods but there are some specific areas of the body that receive direct assistances from higher consumption of these nourishments.

- For a healthy heart: this is the organ that pumps blood throughout the entire body and it gets benefited when we eat strawberries, watermelon, cherries, tomatoes, radishes, beets and peppers.
- For the health of the lungs: this vital organ in our body is benefited when we consume pears, cauliflower, bananas, mushrooms and onions.

- **To have a healthy kidney:** among the foods that help us cleanse the kidneys and our blood are grapes, cabbage, beets, eggplant, plums, grapes and berries.
- **To maintain and improve our digestive health:** our digestive system works best when we eat pineapple, pears, bananas, papaya, kiwi, melon and particularly when we eat fruits and vegetables that are high in natural soluble fiber.
- **For the health of the liver:** the ideal to keep a healthy liver is to eat fruits and vegetables such as spinach, lemon, avocado, cucumber, green grapes, asparagus, beans, broccoli and kiwi.

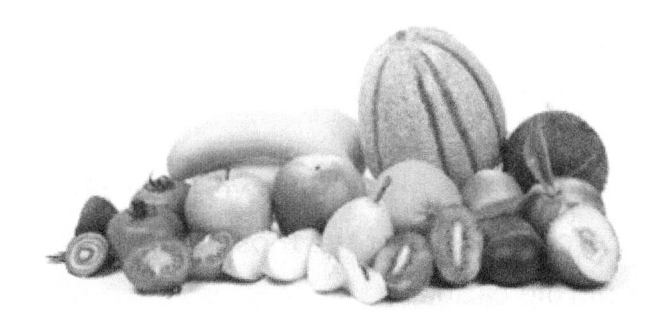

PURPLE CABBAGE: this delicious vegetable is not only good for preparing great salads but also to have a healthier skin.

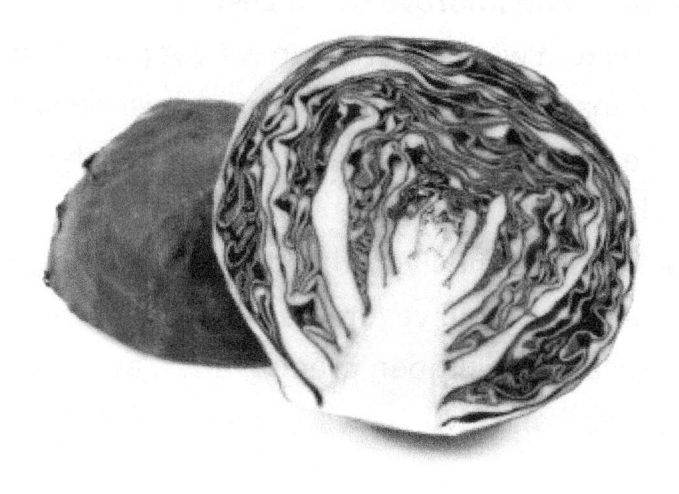

This healthy vegetable also has powerful **antioxidants and vitamins**; here are some of the most important health powers of purple cabbage:

- It has strong anti-inflammatory properties due to its high concentration of abthocyanin **polyphenols**.
- It also has dietary healthy properties due to its antioxidants

- It is good for **reducing the risk of heart disease** according to some studies due to the presence of anthocyanins
- Consuming purple cabbage **is also good for diabetes** and **to prevent certain types of cancer**, it is rich in **vitamin C** and **vitamin K**
- Antioxidants also make your skin look better and younger

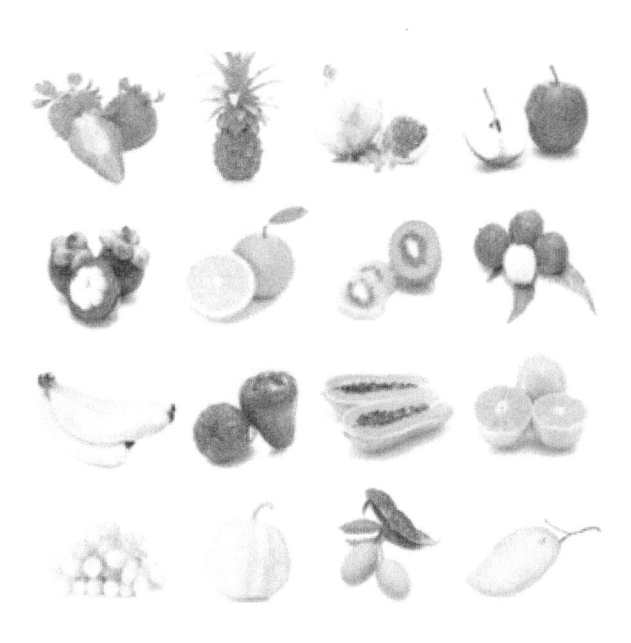

ZUCCHINI: botanically speaking zucchini is considered to be a fruit but it is most commonly known as a vegetable in gastronomic terms. This powerful food is available all year long but the best zucchinis can be found during the summer season or late spring. It has a sweet and delicious flavor that makes it very attractive as a healthy gastronomic option in your daily menu. This delicious fruit **has many nutritional powers** that you can take advantage from if you include it in your menu. Not only it has many health powers but it is also a superfood that is low in calories and high in dietary fiber making it a great choice for those wanting to **lose weight faster** and easier.

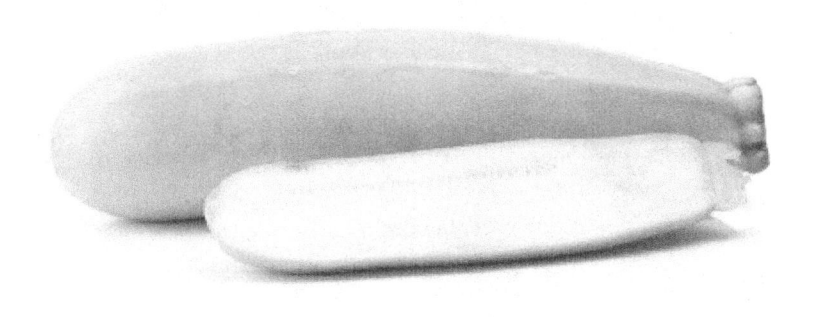

Image courtesy of [Keattikorn] / FreeDigitalPhotos.net

Nutritional Value present in Zucchini

Here is the quantity of nutrients present in 135 gm. of fresh zucchini:

- Calories: 17
- Protein: 1.4 gm.
- Carbohydrate: 3.6 gm.
- Total amount of Fat: 0.17 gm.
- Fiber: 1.5 gm.
- Vitamin C: 11 mg

Here is a list of some of the best health benefits of this powerful fruit:

- Zucchini is a great natural source of phosphorus and magnesium; these two nutrients are crucial for maintaining healthy and strong bones.
- Eating zucchini frequently is great for a low cholesterol diet and to prevent heart disease.
- This marvelous fruit is rich in **vitamin C** and **antioxidants** that can prevent cardiovascular problems naturally.
- It helps protect against oxidation of cells and premature aging thanks to its powerful antioxidants and to a nutrient called beta-carotene.
- When consumed regularly zucchini can help to cleanse your colon due to its dietary fiber and **prevents colon cancer** from occurring.
- Consuming zucchini also helps to maintain a healthier blood vessel system.
- Zucchini is rich in **vitamin B6**, manganese, riboflavin and tons of nutrients.

- This natural food also contains lots of potassium, **vitamin A** and folic acid, all of these essential for adequate body functioning.
- Eating zucchini frequently is also very beneficial for eyes health since it contains lutein and **vitamin C**, both essential for maintaining good healthy eyes.
- This is the perfect healthy snack for people looking to lose weight faster, zucchini is 95% water, **contains natural dietary fiber** and it is low in calories and very high in nutritious value.
- Eating zucchini also helps to cure asthma since it is high in vitamin C levels that also act as a strong antioxidant with **anti-inflammatory properties**.
- Consuming this vegetable-fruit frequently can also help to reducing the risk of having multiple sclerosis.
- This healthy food also helps **to prevent illnesses like bruising and scurvy** that are produced by a deficit in **vitamin C**.

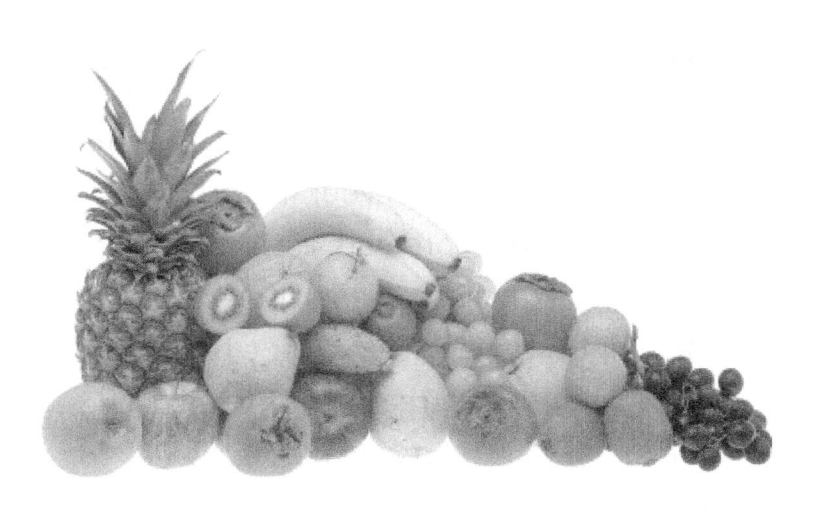

APPLES: in terms of health apple shouldn't be known as the forbidden fruit since it has some very powerful properties that make this healthy food a must have choice in every healthy menu.

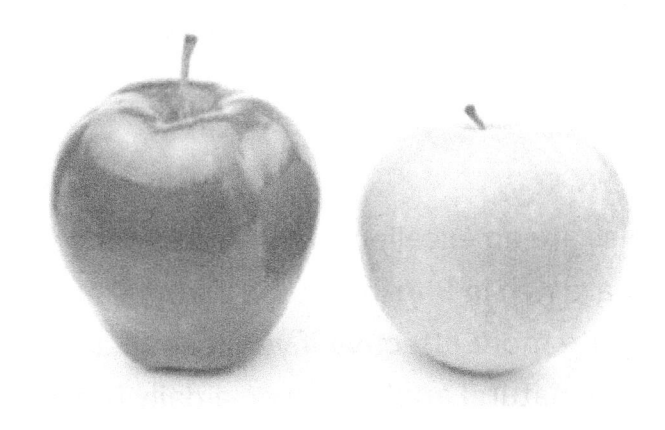

Here is a list of some of the most important benefits of this very healthy fruit:

- If you suffer from frequent headaches than you should include apples in your menu. Taking a ripe apple without the core part of the center of the fruit but only the flesh of the apple in the mornings on an empty stomach with a little bit of **sea salt** is an excellent natural treatment for headaches. You can take this natural recipe during a week to see some good results even if you suffer from major headaches.

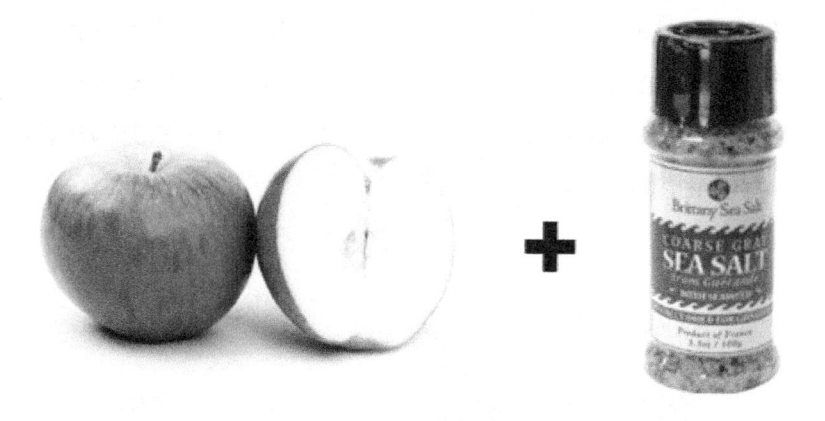

- Apples are an excellent natural cure for anemia; they are rich in Phosphorus, Vitamin C and Iron. They are more effective if you take them in the form of natural apple juice on a daily basis to get good results. You can use a good **juice extractor** to obtain the natural juices of the apple. You can consume this powerful healthy juice 30 minutes prior to taking your meals without adding any refined sugars and 15 minutes before going to bed each day to cure anemia naturally.

- Apple can be used as an effective **natural remedy for stomach illnesses**. The way to use it is to take an entire apple and cut it into slices and then mash the sliced by pounding them until you get a consistent substance. After that you can dust some cinnamon over the mashed apple and eat this as **a great home remedy to cure stomach disorders**. Just keep in mind not to eat the seeds of the apple. Chew this healthy potion before swallowing it. The secret inside this healthy home remedy is the **pectin** present inside the apple that creates a coat protecting the stomach and acts as an absorbent and demulcent with soothing natural and effective properties.

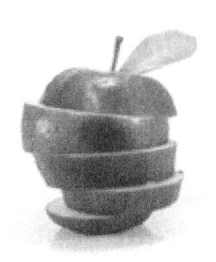

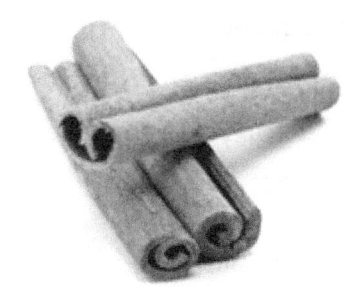

You can also include a healthy preparation of **sliced apples** with some honey and dusted with some sesame seeds in your menu. You can add some lemon also to detox your digestive system. This healthy recipe acts as a powerful **natural stomach tonic** and can be served with any meal as an appetizer or taken as healthy snack during the day.

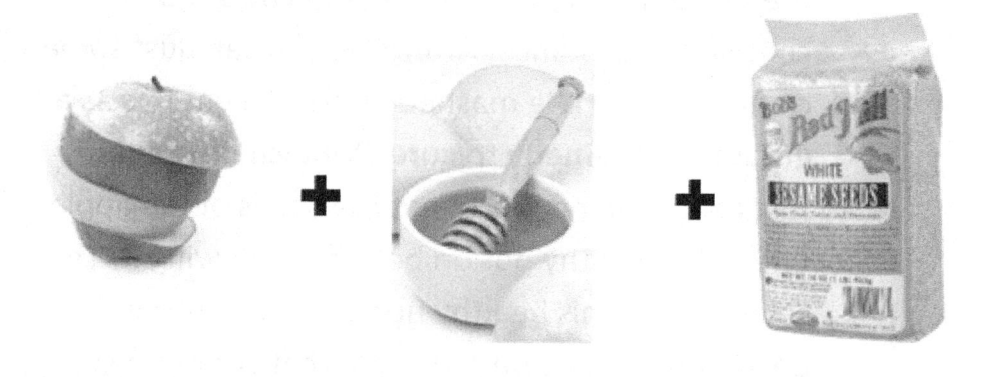

The best and more effective way to take this **fabulous natural remedy** is before meals, by doing this you stimulate your digestive system and then it becomes easier for your stomach to process foods and absorb nutrients.

- Apples are also **great for colon treatment** and for intestinal inflammation (dysentery). A preparation with sweet and ripe crushed apples should be made to treat this type of intestinal illness. The pulp obtained by crushing the apple can be given to small kids suffering from dysentery; the recommended dosage is from 1 to 4 tablespoons during the day. It is e a very effective and natural therapeutic remedy to treat dysentery.

- Apples are also wonderful to treat anemia. This magnificent and delicious fruit is high in nutrients, rich in Iron, Phosphorus and Vitamin C. Taken **in the form of apple juice** it is and excellent home remedy to treat anemia. To get all the benefits the recommended dosage is to drink at least three to four glasses of apple juice per day. You can take this healthy juice just before meals, approximately 30 minutes prior to eating and also before going to sleep. Always prefer **organic apples** and wash them carefully before you put them into your **juice extractor machine.**

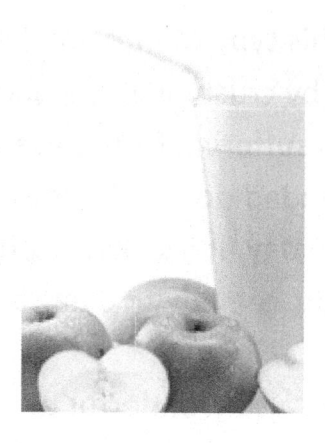

Image courtesy of [NAYPONG] / FreeDigitalPhotos.net

- Apples are also great to treat diarrhea and constipation. Including apples in your daily menu is an all-natural solution for constipation and **to keep a healthy colon**. Take two apples per day to keep doctors away! This will improve your bowel movements since apple is one of the best natural foods containing dietary fiber. Fiber present in apples **makes your digestive system to work better** and your bowel movements will be more frequent **curing constipation**. To treat diarrhea you can eat some cooked apples since the cooking process releases the cellulose inside the apple and makes the stools more consistent. Eating apples frequently will **improve your bowel movements naturally**.

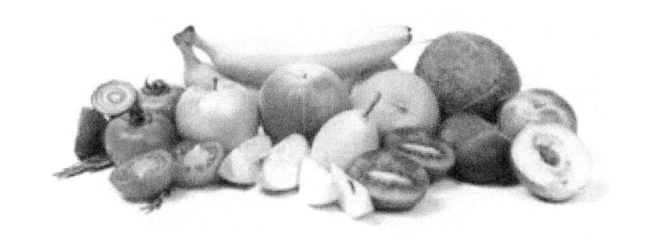

ORANGES: this beautiful fruit has some great benefits and health properties. Oranges, but especially the peel which often times is ignored has excellent properties like helping to lower cholesterol, cut infections, **it helps to fight cancer and also prevents skin cancer**. Some other benefits of this powerful and delicious fruit peel are to act as bug and cat repellent and it is also a very beneficial deodorizer and natural cleanser. The **orange peel** can be used in a number of different ways like added to beverages and deserts when grated. The grated orange peel is also used in a number of different recipes such as muffins and cookies.

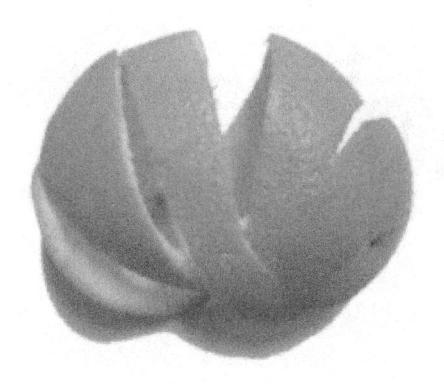

flickr http://www.flickr.com/photos/fdecomite/6298546165/

Here is a list of the benefits you get from consuming the orange peel:

- It is good for lowering bad cholesterol levels naturally. The peel of this wonderful healthy fruit contains a substance called hesperidin, a flavonoid, and also contains polymethoxylated flavones plus pectin. All this ingredients **help to reduce bad cholesterol levels** (LDL levels) naturally and effectively.

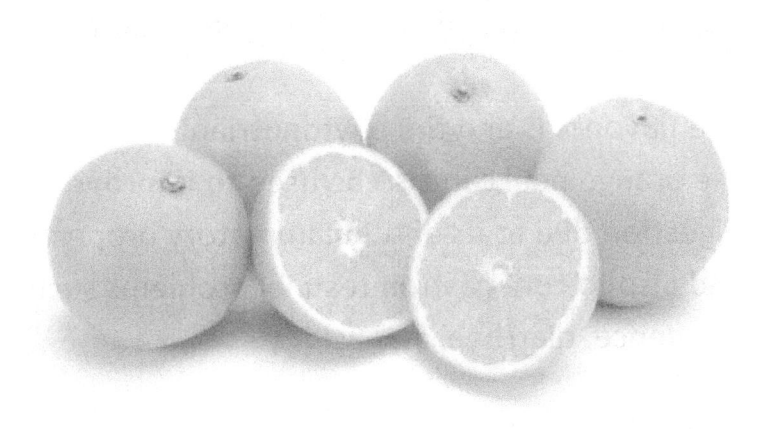

- You can replace chemical repellents with an all-natural option like the orange peel that acts as an effective insect repellent. In order to use the peel for this purpose you must put the peel inside a food processor or blender and pulverizing it. Than you use this peel powder and spread it into your arms or whatever area of your body you want to protect from mosquitoes and other insects without the use of chemicals that only intoxicate your body. You can also use the oil from the peel as a repellent when applied directly into your skin. You can also use it to repel cats since they don´t like the strong smell of the orange peel. Additionally being acid gives the orange peel cleansing properties and it can be used as an effective deodorizer too. Some household cleaners and products like soap use it as a powerful ingredient for cleaning and for aromatization.

- The flavonoids and the phytonutrients present in the orange peel can also be used **to improve digestion** due to its anti-inflammatory properties and also to cure gastrointestinal problems such as flatulence, diarrhea, and acidity.

- It is also great **to treat breast cancer** and to fight bone loss due to the presence of the hesperidin ingredient contained in the orange peel that has anti-inflammatory properties when consumed frequently. Another ingredient present in the orange peel, d-lemonade, can act as protection against ultraviolet rays making this natural ingredient an excellent sunscreen that helps to prevent skin cancer. It can be applied into the skin directly by rubbing it against the area you want to protect or it can also be added to lotions and skin oils. When used topically orange peel can **cure acne**, pimples, wrinkles and premature aging and it can also be used for healthy skin baths with the added benefit of an invigorating scent.

- Orange peel has strong **antioxidant properties** that improve your immune system with its **vitamin A** and **vitamin C**. These properties make it an excellent choice for preventing infections, preventing colds and flu.

- Oranges are also rich in dietary fiber and full of nutrients. It is an excellent natural food for effective excess body weight treatment since it contains pectin and fiber. Pectin has natural laxative properties and also helps to detoxify our bodies by protecting the mucous membrane of the colon acting as a healthy coat that protects against toxic substances.

- Eating oranges also helps to detox our bodies due to a diversity of phytochemicals inside this powerful superfood like Hesperetin and Narigenin. These substances are flavonoids found in citrus fruits and they act as powerful **antioxidants** that fight free radicals.

- It helps to control heart rate thanks to minerals like potassium and calcium. Potassium is an essential component of cell and body fluids that **helps to control blood pressure** and heart rate naturally.

- Drinking an **orange juice** first thing in the morning has many health benefits like detoxifying your body and giving your system important nutrients and vitamins to energize your body. Take a glass of fresh organic orange juice every morning to improve your health without adding any refined sugars. One glass of fresh orange juice has approximately 120 mg of **vitamin C**

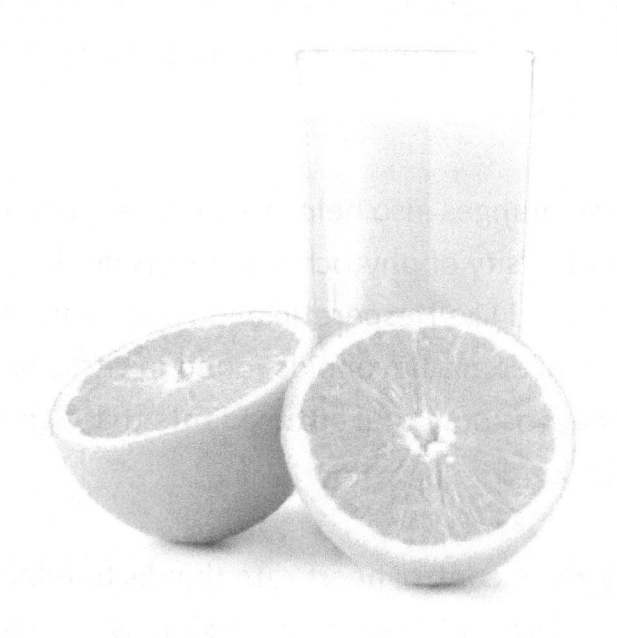

PEACHES: this fruit has many advantages like being low in calories and high in fiber, a great choice for those wanting to lose weight fast. This is a delicious fruit that is easy to digest and also great to improve your digestive system. It has natural laxative properties and **diuretic properties** as well, great for those with urinary tract issues. Eating peaches helps to detox your kidneys and gallbladder naturally. When you eat peaches bile production increases so your digestion improves and it is easier to process fats and other foods.

Peaches also contain **phosphorus**; this is an essential component for a healthy brain and a healthy nervous system. Consuming peaches is great for managing stress levels, fatigue and anxiety thanks to the magnesium it contains. Taking peach in the form of natural juice is also great to dissolve kidney stones naturally and effectively. Consuming this fruit frequently also helps to prevent constipation thank to its great quantity of dietary fiber.

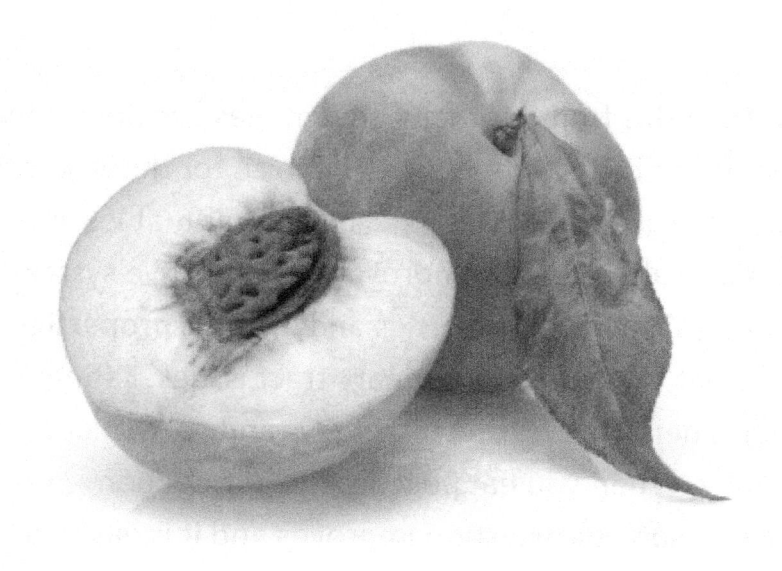

On top of having a great flavor, peaches have powerful antioxidant properties; they contain lots of **vitamin A, vitamin C and vitamin E** that help to prevent premature aging and the decay of tissue. Due to its antioxidants it is also great to consume peaches to prevent degenerative diseases such as Alzheimer, cataracts and cancer. **Potassium** and vitamin A also have a great influence on your system improving heart rate, improving vision and also preventing gastrointestinal infections. It is also great to improve your skin health and a great natural provider of energy. Peaches have a great percentage of water (85% approx.) and are low in calories.

PEARS: this very juicy and delicious fruit also has some great health qualities and benefits. Here are some of the most important health benefits of pears:

- Consuming pears frequently helps to prevent premature aging and prevents macular degeneration.
- Including pears on your daily menu is great for your colon health and your digestive system health, this one of the top fruit choices when it comes to high fiber foods. **Eating high fiber foods is essential for your colon health,** fiber is not digested and acts a as a broom inside your intestine cleaning all toxins and excess fat trapped in the colon walls. It also improves bowel movements and prevents and cures constipation.

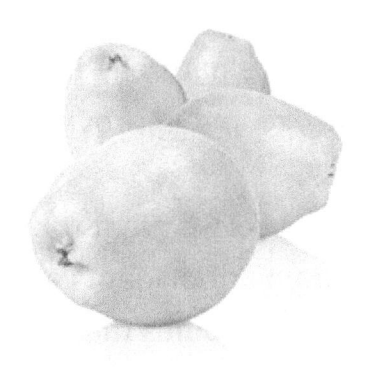

- Eating pears is an excellent choice to improve your immune system due to the powerful antioxidants this yummy fruit contains.
- It is a great choice for pregnant women since it prevents neural tube defects in infants.
- Consumed in the form of natural juice it also has great health benefits like helping **to reduce pain in many inflammatory problems**.
- Consuming pears is great for bones health since they contain boron to help your body to keep calcium.
- It also helps to lower bad cholesterol levels thanks to the high amounts of pectin it contains.
- Pears are a magnificent and healthy source of energy since they contain fructose and glucose, especially in the form of organic juice.
- Pear juice may also help **to reduce fever naturally**.
- Eating pears regularly is also very helpful to reduce high blood pressure naturally therefore reducing the risk of a stroke and improving your heart health.
- Consuming pears is also great for your cells health since they contain antioxidants and **vitamin C**.
- According to some studies the inclusion of pears in a healthy diet for women is very beneficial to prevent postmenopausal breast cancer.

Some of the nutrients present in pears are: vitamin B6, vitamin C, Calcium, Magnesium, Zinc, Iron, Phosphorus, Folate, Niacin, vitamin B5, dietary fiber, Thiamin, Protein, Riboflavin, natural sugars and carbohydrates.

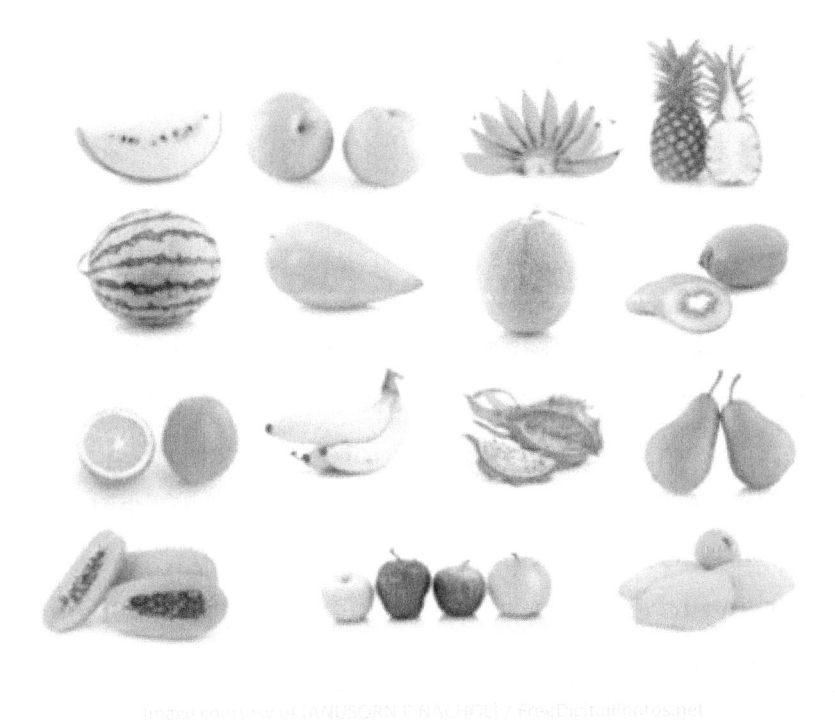

BLACKBERRIES: this is one of the fruits with the highest amounts of antioxidants. This aspect alone gives this fruit very powerful health property like reduce the risk of many types of cancer like breast cancer and gastrointestinal cancer.

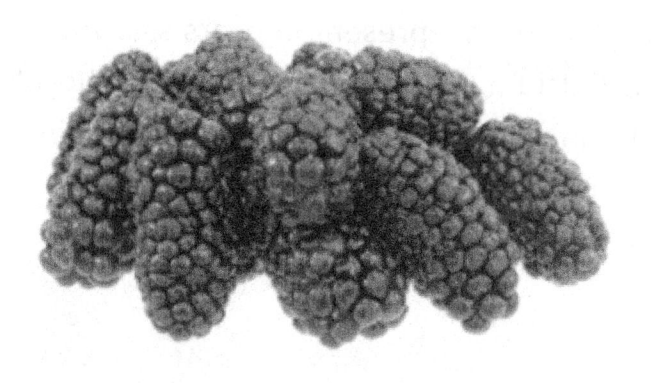

The antioxidant substance present in blackberries is called anthocyanin and it helps to boost collagen production, it also stops swelling and it also improves circulation. Another powerful substance contained in this great fruit is Folate, an essential vitamin to prevent many forms of cancer and to ease the risk of Alzheimer's disease.

By eating blackberries regularly you also prevent the risk of heart disease due to the presence of **Omega 3 fatty acids**. Also Omega-3 fatty acids are recognized for its ability to improve brain function and the performance of memory. Blackberries are also loaded with beneficial and essential vitamins like vitamin A and vitamin K. You can supply half of your body's needed daily vitamin C dosage just by consuming blackberries and get almost 35% of the vitamin K your body needs for the day. Be sure to eat only organic blackberries and ripe blackberries to get all the benefits and stay away from pesticides and harmful chemicals.

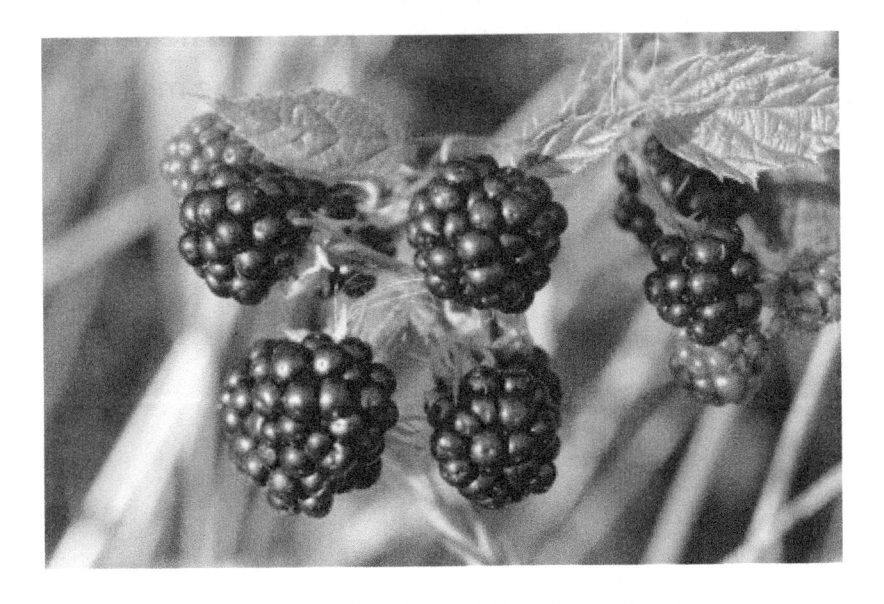

Blackberries are also an excellent choice **to fortify blood vessels** and to help recover eyesight. They contain a substance called tannin that helps to tighten tissue, alleviate intestinal inflammation and helps to cure hemorrhoids and stomach illnesses. Consuming this tiny fruit frequently also may help to prevent the risk of developing diabetes according to some studies. They can be taken during the day as a very healthy snack both by adults and kids.

STRAWBERRIES: on top of being one of the most beautiful and sexy fruits out there and also having aphrodisiac properties, strawberries are high in essential **healthy nutrients and vitamins.** Here are some of the most important powers and health benefits you get from the consumption of this delicious fruit:

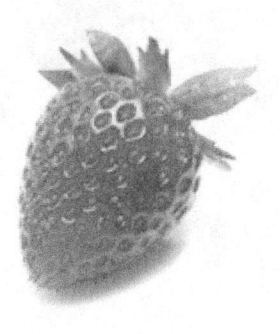

Image courtesy of [MASTER ISOLATED IMAGES] / FreeDigitalPhotos.net

- You **improve your immune system** when you eat strawberries. By taking just 1 cup of this magnificent red fruit you get more of the recommended daily dosage of vitamin C that your body needs to stay healthy. **Vitamin C** present in this fruit can also help you to reduce blood pressure naturally and effectively. Its powerful **antioxidants** are also great to fight macular degeneration and cataracts. Vitamin C is also good to give strength to the cornea and retina.

- Strawberries contain a substance that is very beneficial for bones health, this substance is Manganese. This fruit is also great for kids to maintain adequate bone development and bone strength. Bones are also nourished by the **vitamin K**, the magnesium and the potassium present in strawberries.

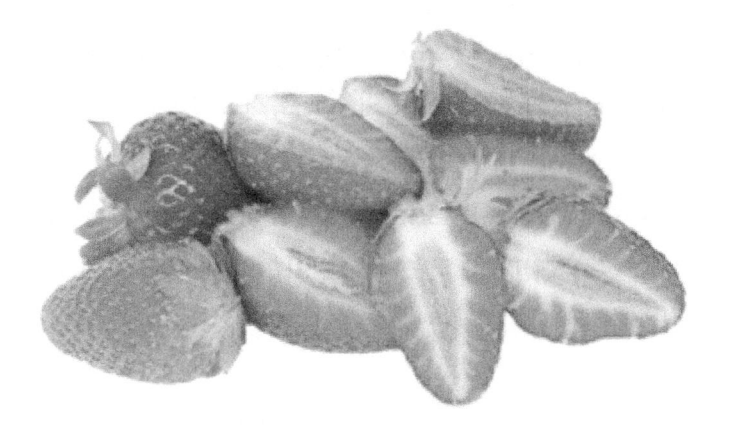

- Recent studies have shown that by eating strawberries frequently the risk of eye age related diseases like macular degeneration is greatly reduced.

- Anti-inflammatory properties and **antioxidant properties** present on strawberries helps to fight against the appearance of different types of cancer.

Folate, vitamin C, flavonoids quercetin and kaemplerol constitute a great natural shield that protects human cells against cancer development.

- To fight inflammatory illnesses like atherosclerosis, asthma, and osteoarthritis it is recommended to include strawberries on your daily menu. They contain a natural **anti-inflammatory agent** called phenols that fights against these diseases. It acts by blocking the enzyme cyclooxygenase (COX) just as some chemical based drugs like aspirin or ibuprofen do. Always prefer natural alternatives over chemical solutions to detox your body naturally.

- Eating strawberries is also a great solution for those wanting to detox their bodies naturally. Just 1 cup of strawberries contains enough **manganese to fight cellular inflammation preventing heart disease** and manganese is also a powerful natural antioxidant.

- Eating strawberries regularly is also excellent for dieting. This is **one of the fruits with the highest amount of dietary fiber** with one cup containing over 14% of the recommended daily dosage of fiber and with low calories, just 42 calories approximately per serving.

- The red color in this magical and powerful fruit is due to an antioxidant substance called Anthocyanin. These phenols antioxidant substances make this fruit a great powerful superfood that should be part of everybody´s menu to prevent premature aging and to detoxify your system naturally.

- Vitamin C in strawberries also **stimulates the natural production of collagen** and improves the look and the elasticity of your skin naturally.

- Eating strawberries regularly is great **to reduce bad cholesterol levels**. The presence of phytochemicals like ellagic and flavonoids inside this wonderful fruit help to fight bad cholesterol levels and also improve your heart health preventing the buildup of plaque in the arteries.

- Including strawberries in a healthy diet is a great strong alternative for women who are pregnant. They contain folate, a vitamin recommended for women who are pregnant. Folate is essential for a healthy development of the baby´s brain and also the folic acid contained in strawberries may help to prevent birth defects.

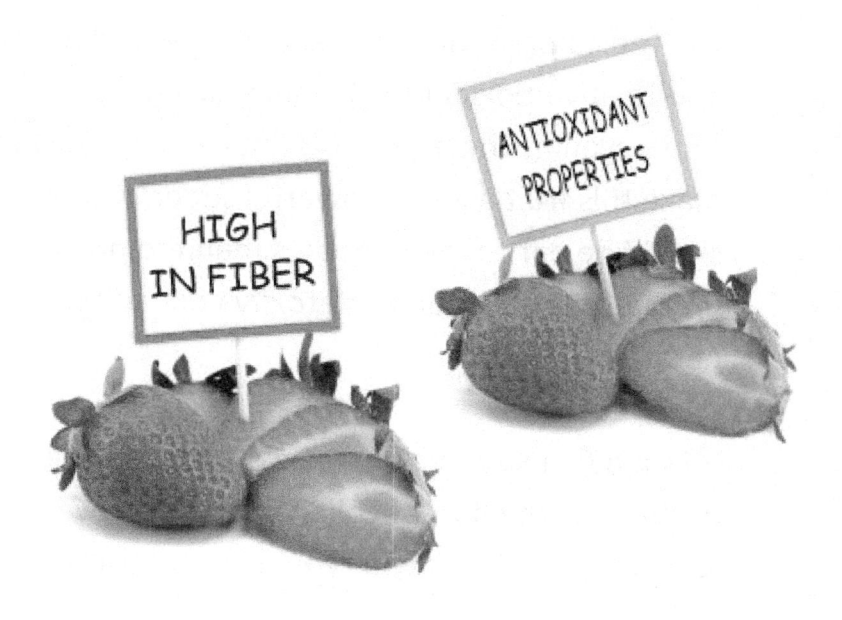

GRAPES: if you want to have a healthy and strong life than you have to include grapes in your diet. This wonderful fruit has multiple health benefits like curing the lack of energy, curing kidney conditions, it is good for indigestion, and it cures constipation and also prevents macular degeneration and prevents the appearance of cataracts. Here is a list of the most important benefits you get when you consume this fruit on a regular basis:

- **Resveratrol** present in grapes is an excellent natural ingredient that reduces the levels of amyloidal-beta peptides in patients with Alzheimer's disease. According to some serious studies and researches consuming grapes can **improve brains health** notably and prevent some neurological diseases naturally and effectively.

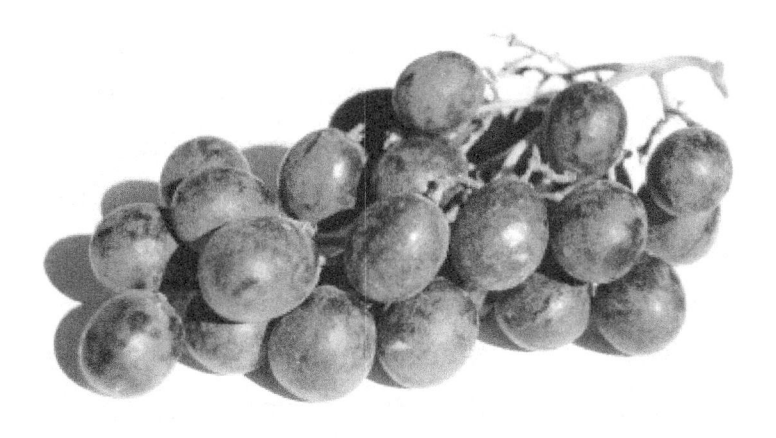

- If you are looking to reduce your cholesterol levels naturally then you must include this fruit on your menu. Grapes have a substance called pterostilbene that has the ability **to bring bad cholesterol levels down**. The skin of this fruit can also help you to lower your cholesterol levels since it contains saponin that prevents the absorption of bad cholesterol.

- Eating grapes frequently is a great natural alternative **to prevent macular degeneration**. It can greatly diminish the risk of this degenerative eyes disease if consumed on a regular basis.

- Grapes are a great natural superfood that has powerful **anti-cancer benefits** thanks to the anti-inflammatory properties of **resveratrol** contained in this fruit. Some of the substances inside grapes like **proanthocyanidins** and **anthocyanins** have anti-proliferation properties that constrain the proliferation of cancer cells. Also consuming grapes can **boost the strength of your immune system**.

- Speaking of immunity system regular consumption of red grapes has powerful **antiviral and antibacterial properties** and is excellent **to fight infections**. Grapes have robust antiviral properties that fight poliovirus and herpes simplex virus.

- Eating grapes also helps **to prevent the appearance of cataracts** thanks to the flavonoids it contains that are powerful natural antioxidants. This

antioxidants decrease the harm caused by free radicals like cancer, cardiovascular diseases, premature aging and cataracts.

- Consuming grapes can **improve kidney conditions** by eliminating uric acid from the system naturally and effectively.

- Grapes are great to maintain and improve energy levels naturally due to the iron they contain. It has a **great energy boosting effect** when consumed in the form of **juice**.

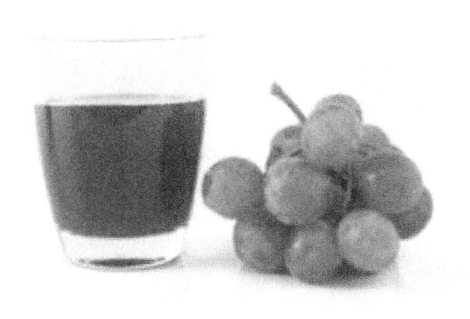

- Another health benefit of grapes is that they are excellent **to treat constipation** and act as a natural laxative due to the organic acid they contain. They

provide relieve from chronic constipation by **relaxing the intestine**.
- Grapes are great for curing the irritated stomach and also as a natural remedy for indigestion.

CHERRIES: cherries are one of the top fruits when it comes to fiber amounts. They are among the most powerful fruits in terms of health benefits. Here are some of the best and more beneficial properties of eating cherries:

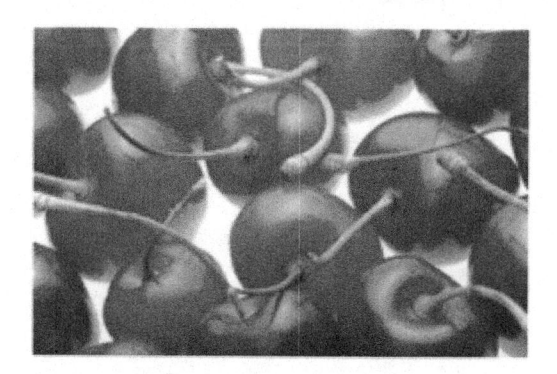

Image courtesy of [ZOLE4] / FreeDigitalPhotos.net

- They are great **to reduce the risk of diabetes**.
- They can be taken as a healthy snack at any time during the day to maintain a slim body

- Consuming cherries is also great to ease joint pain and soreness for athletes and runners alike due to its powerful **anti-inflammatory properties**.
- They are an **excellent source of dietary fiber** that helps the colon health, the proper function of the digestive system and are great for those looking to lose weight fast.
- Cherries are a great source of energy; they contain iron, vitamin C, vitamin E, potassium, folate and magnesium.
- This fruit has an impressive amount of beta carotene (vitamin A), they have as much as 19 times more beta carotene that other fruits like strawberries or blueberries. **Beta carotene enhances immunity** and also improves your skin condition.
- Eating cherries is **great for your brain** and it is an excellent natural food to prevent the loss of memory.
- Eating cherries is **good for inflammatory problems** like arthritis and gout.
- Cherries are **great for your heart´s health** since they contain melatonin, a healthy antioxidant that is beneficial for the proper functioning of the heart and the natural regulation of heart rhythm and also body sleep cycles.

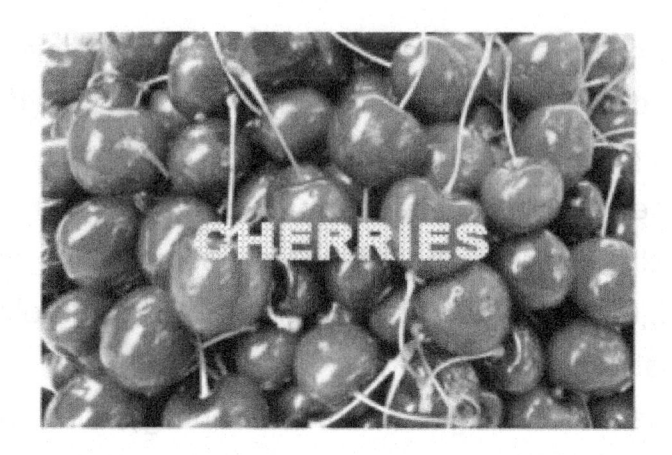

Image courtesy of [NTWOWE] / FreeDigitalPhotos.net

- Cherry is considered a **superfood** and it is **full of antioxidants** called anthocyanins that help to reduce the risk of a stroke and reduces the chances of having cancer.

WATER MELON: this healthy food is not only very refreshing but also packed with powerful nutrients and vitamins. It is a strong natural source of antioxidants. Here is a list of the best health benefits this wonderful and delicious juicy fruit has to offer:

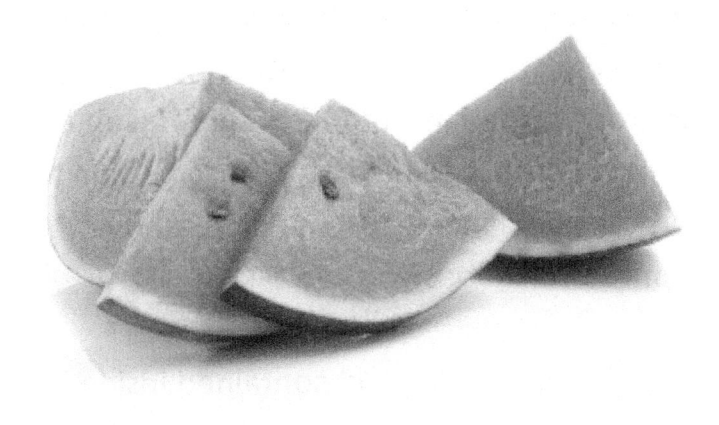

- It helps to **reduce asthma** due to its antioxidants. It is an excellent fruit to consume **to decrease the risk of heart disease**, prostate cancer and rheumatoid arthritis.

- Eating watermelon helps to **prevent macular degeneration**; this wonderful fruit contains beta carotene, vitamin C, Lutein and Zeaxanthin, all these antioxidant ingredients that will protect your eyes health.

- Eating water melon is an excellent natural alternative **to treat impotence**. An ingredient present in this delicious watery fruit called **Arginine** is great **to improve blood circulation** and to promote **Nitric Oxide** natural production **to boost erections**. In fact water melon is among the best aphrodisiac foods you can take.

- Lypocene, a carotenoid contained inside water melon is great for **improving heart functions**. Also the **beta carotene** found in this fruit is an excellent anti-oxidant that prevents premature aging and keeps your heart in a healthy and strong condition. The carotenoids and the potassium in water melon **reduce the risk of heart attack** by **reducing levels of bad cholesterol** at the same time.

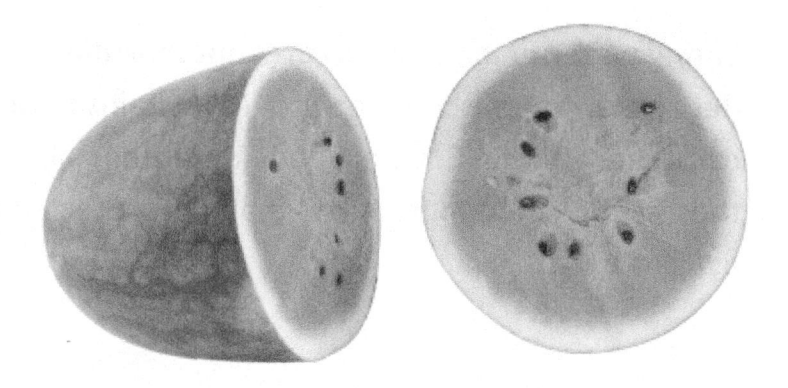

- Water Melons are a great natural and healthy supplement for patients with diabetes that are in a low sugar diet. Although this delicious and **refreshing fruit** is sweet in taste it is very **low in calories** since almost all the fruit is composed of water and roughage. It also contains numerous vitamins and **nutrients like potassium and magnesium** that promotes proper functioning of insulin in your system by lowering the blood sugar levels at the same time. Another ingredient contained in water melons, the **Arginine** promotes the healthy impact of insulin on sugar.

- Water Melon is a very refreshing natural food and it is high in citrulline that stimulates the arginine in our bodies that helps our system to get rid of ammonia.

- Water Melon contains **lycopene**; this powerful antioxidant gives this fruit its red characteristics and also helps our bodies **to fight free radicals**. It is also great for **preventing many types of cancers** like lung cancer, prostate cancer and stomach cancer.

Lycopene also **promotes heart health** and it reinforces the immune system. It can also be found in the form of natural supplements.

BANANAS: on top of being a delicious fruit with aphrodisiac properties, bananas have tons of health benefits. It is a great idea to include bananas in your daily menu if you want to strengthen your overall health. This is one of the fruits with the most nutrients and vitamins that we can find in nature; in fact they have **more health benefits than apples** so it can be fair to say that one banana a day will do the trick of keeping doctor away instead of one apple a day. Bananas have 5 times as much **vitamin A** and iron then apples and they also contain 3 times more phosphorus making them **a real natural superfood!** Here are some of the greatest health benefits of bananas:

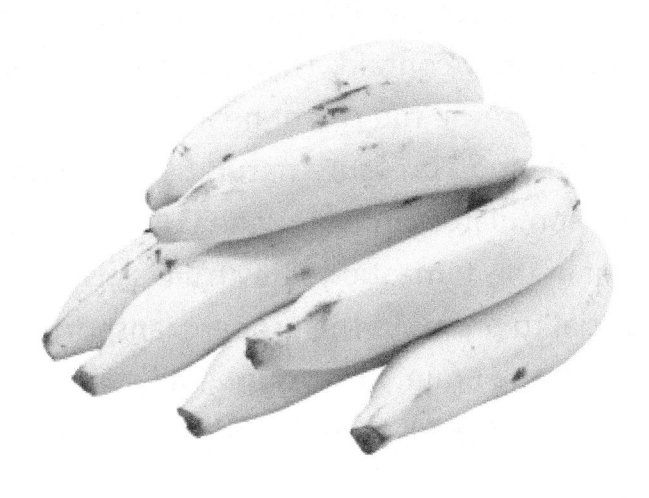

- Bananas are **a great source of natural energy** due to the high amounts of vitamins and minerals they contain. Just by eating 2 bananas before a workout you will give your body all the energy it needs. They are also a great natural snack to take whenever you are feeling tired or without the energy to keep going. It is a great and healthier alternative to taking caffeine with refine sugars that will give you a much longer lasting **effect of extra energy** without the crash caused when you consume caffeine products.

- One of the key elements of bananas is the **potassium** they contain. This powerful ingredient helps to decrease the risk of heart attacks and also to **control blood pressure naturally** and effectively since it stimulates circulatory health. The potassium present in this fantastic yellow fruit is also beneficial to promote the proper transportation of oxygen to the brain. **Potassium** is a key ingredient for great body performance and to maintain a healthy heart rate and a good balance of water in your system.

- Eating bananas frequently also **promotes adequate and healthy bowel movements** preventing and curing constipation naturally. This is one of the fruits with the highest concentration of dietary fiber beneficial for proper digestion.

- Eating bananas is **great to relieve stress** and depression symptoms naturally without the use of drugs. They contain a substance called tryptophan that **helps to regulate your mood naturally** relaxing your mind by keeping away stress feelings and mood swings. The **vitamin B6** present in bananas also is very helpful in regulating blood glucose levels in your system thus helping to improve your mood.

- They can help you **to reduce the effect of a hangover** due to its natural restoring abilities. When you eat bananas your body receives a ton of nutrients that restore your system **reducing the effects of a hangover** naturally. One great recipe to achieve this restoring effect is to mix two bananas in a blender with a yogurt and some honey and drink this healthy potion to get all the benefits. This powerful blend heals your stomach and with the honey your blood sugar levels are restored. Another great benefit of eating bananas is for those who are trying to quit smoking since they counteract against the addictive effects of nicotine.

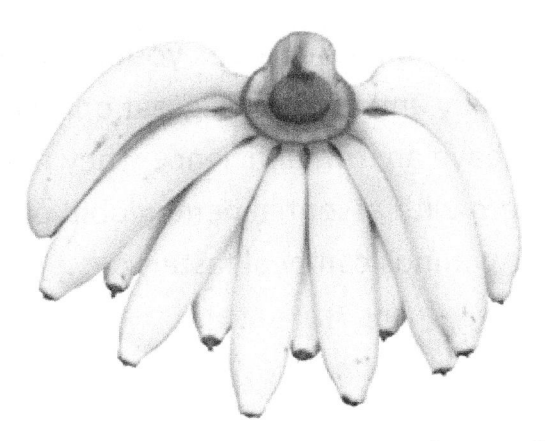

- According to some studies eating bananas can **improve brain functions** naturally especially in kids. The study found that kids eating bananas once a day during breakfast were more attentive during the different learning sessions at school.

- Among the many benefits you can get from bananas there is one that may surprise you and that is that you can **use them as a natural mosquito bite healing agent**. You can use the peel of the banana and rub the inside of it on your skin to ease the itching and swelling caused by mosquito bites. This is definitively a better option to cure and alleviate mosquito bites than the chemical based medications you get at the drugstore.

- Eating bananas **increases your energy levels naturally** and they are a great option for people that have an **iron** deficiency. They provide your system with essential hemoglobin production so your wounds can heal faster.

- Consuming bananas is great **to heal stomach ulcers** since they reduce the acidity that some foods have causing gastrointestinal problems. When you eat bananas **your digestive system benefits** from a shielding coating provided by this wonderful fruit so you ease internal irritation. If you suffer from heartburn eating bananas is a great natural solution due to their capacity to offset stomach acidity. So instead of taking pharmaceutical antacids you can eat bananas and rapidly calm the stomach burn.

- Bananas are a great natural alternative **to get rid of warts**. You can use the outside of the peel and put it on warts to make them disappear. You can use some kind of tape to keep the banana peel in place against the wart you want to eliminate.

  If you want to keep doctor and visits to the hospital as far as you can than you have to start eating this yellow magic fruit as frequently as you can to get all the health benefits of bananas.

By eating just one banana a day your immune system gets a powerful boost!

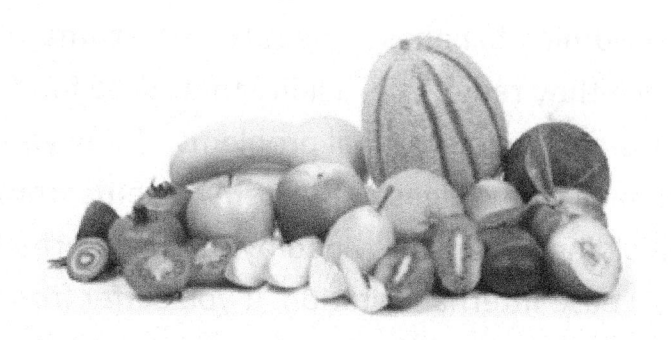

Eat Well and Stay Healthy!

MANGOSTEEN: this delicious and exotic fruit provides many health benefits. Many serious studies have demonstrated the benefits of consuming this fruit. One of the main reasons of why Mangosteen is so beneficial is because it has in excess of forty natural chemical compounds called Xanthones. Among these many biologically-active ingredients contained inside this wonderful super fruit you can benefit from powerful antioxidants like Alpha-mangostin. Another powerful antioxidant present in this fruit is the Gamma-mangostin that acts as a strong anti-inflammatory agent. Eating mangosteen on a frequent basis is also great **to fight tumors** due to another powerful antioxidant present in this fruit called Garcione E.

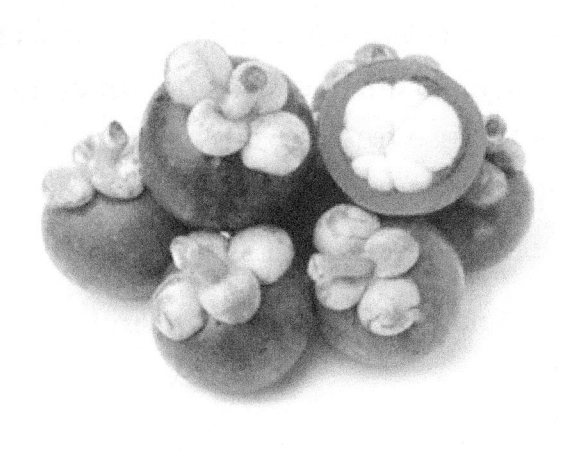

A very large number of diseases can be prevented and even treated while consuming mangosteen. For ages Asian cultures have recognized the healing powers of this magical and exotic fruit and its many benefits. Among the many uses of this fruit we can find the following: they help to cure inflammatory problems naturally, stop infection and boost energy naturally. Many studies have also found the amazing properties of the fruit **to prevent some diseases like Alzheimer´s disease**, many types of cancers, diabetes and heart disease among others. When Queen Victoria stated that she liked this fruit it was named the "Queen of Fruits".

Mangosteens contain Xanthones; this antioxidant **protects our bodies against free radicals**, different viruses, has anti-fungal properties and boosts our immune system naturally. Free radicals make our bodies to age sooner than it should and weakens our immune system. So to neutralize these free radicals we must consume fruits rich in antioxidants like mangosteens. Antioxidants help to <u>detox our bodies naturally</u> and effectively.

Other powerful natural ingredients present in the Mangosteen fruit:

> Other powerful components inside mangosteens include polysaccharides, polyphenols, catechins, quinones and stilbenes.

> If you want all the power of **Vitamin C** multiplied by 5 then you have to choose to consume mangosteens on a regular basis. Also among the most powerful anti-cancer agents you can find in nature are the

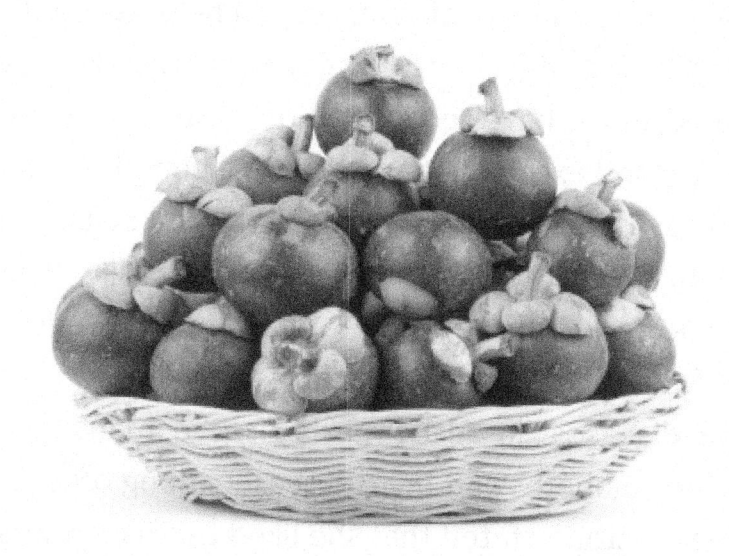

polysaccharides found inside this marvelous fruit. This powerful ingredient also has strong **antibacterial properties** like a substance called quinones also present in this magical and wonderful fruit. Stilbenes, another strong antioxidant that mangosteens contain have **anti-fungal properties**. One of the amazing things about this fruit is that its **polyphenols** are much stronger as an antioxidant than **vitamin E.**

You can take mangosteen in the form of **juice** to get all the health benefits it has. Here is a list of the powers of this great fruit:

- It has powerful antifungal properties and helps to stop fungal infections
- Eating mangosteens is great **to stop premature aging**
- Mangosteens have anti-arthritic properties
- It is great to prevent bacterial infections
- It has anti-allergic properties
- Eating mangosteens is great **to prevent arthritis**
- Great anti-inflammatory properties can be found in this fruit
- It works as a **natural anti-depressant**
- Helps to control your nervous system naturally
- Eating this fruit regularly increases your energy levels naturally

- Helps to prevent atherosclerotic problems and the hardening of arteries
- It also helps to **prevent the appearance of kidney stones**
- Helps to treat diarrhea
- Helps to prevent the appearance of glaucoma
- It has anti-cataract properties
- Helps to regulate the neurological system
- Helps to reduce obesity problems and it is good for natural weight loss
- It helps **to prevent the appearance of tumors**
- It helps to prevent the appearance of Parkinson's disease
- It helps to strengthen your bones and acts as a natural anti-osteoporosis agent
- It helps **to reduce fever naturally**
- Consuming mangosteens helps to avoid dizziness
- It avoids viral infections
- It helps to fight anxiety
- It **strengthens your immune system**
- It controls healthy blood pressure
- It stabilizes sugar levels in your system

You can get all the benefits from this great fruit [buying it online](#) or consuming it in the form of healthy mangosteen juice.

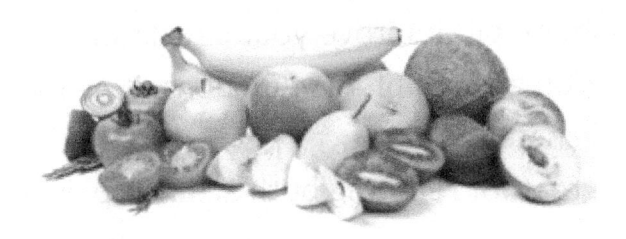

"Using lots of fresh foods, fruits and vegetables, helps to keep the menu buoyant - I don't know if that's the right word, but it keeps a balance of freshness and health." - Sally Schneider

MANDARINS: mandarin also known as tangerine is a delicious citrus fruit with tons of health beneficial properties. Tangerine essential oil has powerful therapeutic properties. This oil is obtained from the mandarin peel and contains many beneficial substances for our health. Here is a list of the benefits of mandarin essential oils:

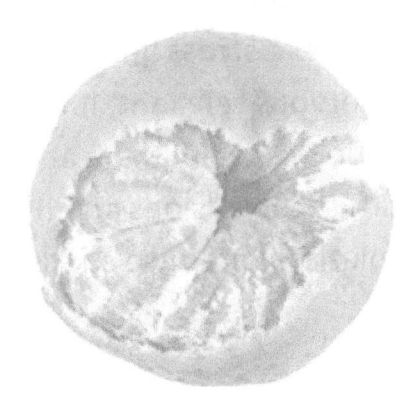

- Mandarin oils improve your circulatory system function and lymphatic functions. It helps to rejuvenate the skin.
- It is great for relieving both arthritis pain and rheumatism and it enhances your immunity system.
- **It has beneficial digestive properties**, just a few drops of mandarin oil after meals improves digestion notably by stimulating the digestive juices in your stomach.
- This powerful natural oil also acts as a **very good tonic stimulating the respiratory system**, the neurological system, the endocrinal system and the circulatory system naturally.
- It has hepatic properties, **mandarin oil is great for the liver´s health** and it promotes the effective discharge of bile and keeps infections away. It is great to strengthen the liver.
- It is **great to relieve stress** and act as a powerful and **natural nervous relaxant**. It has a southing and relaxing sedation capacity that can even calm epilepsy attacks, convulsions and hysteria. It is an all-natural solution to reduce stress.

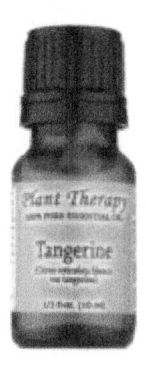

- It protects the stomach from ulcers and other stomach illnesses like infections.
- It is great for treating constipation, diarrhea, and flatulence and **improves the digestive system function**.
- It is great to treat scars and any type of skin marks like stretch marks.
- It also helps to detox your body naturally by getting rid of toxic waste through urine, sweat or through excretion.
- It **promotes the rapid healing of wounds** by stimulating the growth of tissue and new cells.
- It is **beneficial for the respiratory system** and also has antiseptic properties protecting wounds from infection and bacteria by forming a protective shield on the wound.
- Mandarin oil has **anti spasmodic powers** and it is great to cure muscular spasms and digestive system

spasms, just a few drops will give you the relieve you need naturally and effectively.

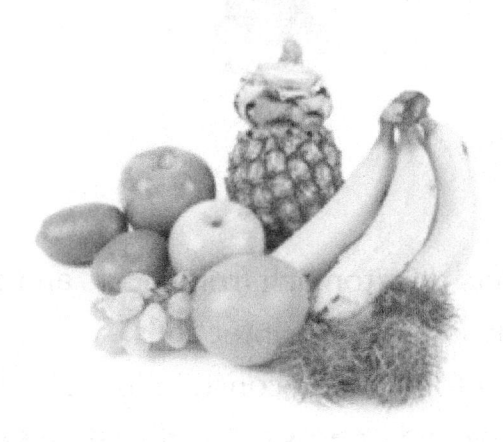

"Foods high in bad fats, sugar and chemicals are directly linked to many negative emotions, whereas whole, natural foods rich in nutrients - foods such as fruits, vegetables, grains and legumes - contribute to greater energy and positive emotions." - Marilu Henner

LEMONS: since ancient Egyptians the powerful properties of lemons have been recognized. This powerful acid fruit has many wonderful properties like acting as a powerful natural antibacterial, a powerful immune system booster, and antiviral properties. **It also has cleansing properties to detox your liver naturally** and it is also great for weight loss for its digestive benefits. Inside lemons we can find a number of very beneficial substances like pectin, bioflavonoids, magnesium, calcium and of course citric acid that gives this wonderful its antiseptic properties. Here is a list of other healing powers of lemons:

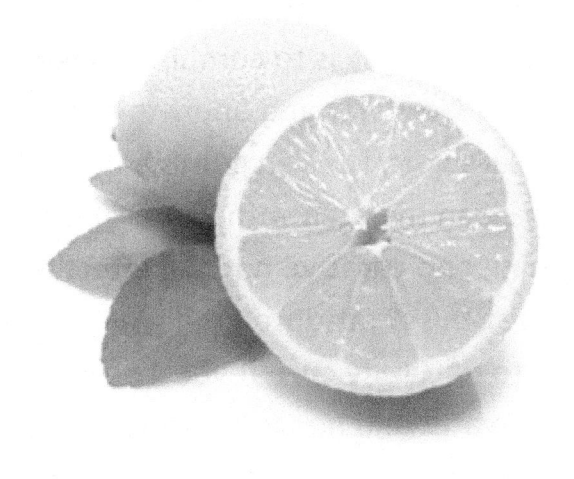

- **Including lemons in your diet is a great natural remedy to fight fatigue**. According to some studies consuming lemons frequently has a relaxing effect on your nervous system. Inhalation lemon oil can boost your concentration levels and also reduces fatigue and anxiety.
- Lemon is great to treat acne problems due to the citric acid it contains. Your skin benefits from the high amounts of **vitamin C** found in lemons that helps **to eliminate bacteria causing acne**. One great habit to adopt is to drink a glass of water with lemon first thing in the morning to detox your

system and to keep your skin clean. You can also apply a few drops of lemon juice directly on acne to see the results. Another mix that you can use to treat acne naturally is to combine squeezed lemon juice with rose water and apply this mixture on the affected area of your skin gently. After 30 minutes you can clean the area with water and this will have a **soothing and curative natural effect on acne**. You can repeat this procedure until you see the results.

- It helps **to naturally cure fever**. You can drink it with hot water and honey and a few drops of lemon as a natural remedy to cure fever. Ideally you should add the juice of one entire lemon to the hot water and drink this healing potion at once. Repeat every two hours approximately until the fever disappears.
- Lemons are an excellent natural cure **to treat the flu**. Loaded with vitamin C consuming lemons are both great to prevent the flu and to treat it naturally. It gives your immune system a natural boost and helps to get rid of viruses. Drinking natural lemon juice frequently is one of the best immune boosters your body can take. To cure sore throat symptoms you can prepare a healthy beverage that consists of lemon juice with 1 tablespoon of sea salt with warm water. You can do gargles approximately three times during the day

with this healthy potion to get the relieve you need. The **antibacterial and antiviral properties** of lemon will do the magic.

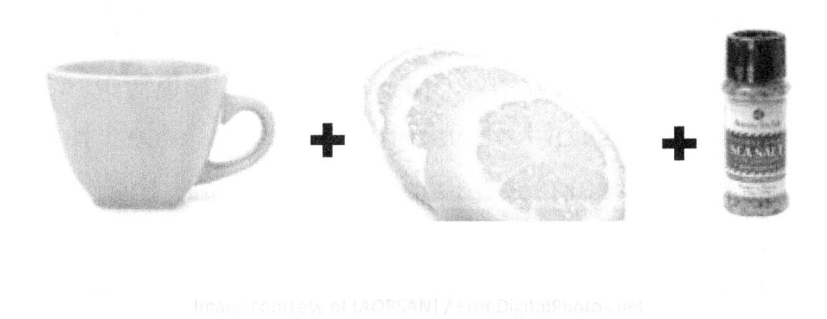

- Drinking lemon juice is an excellent natural energy booster that helps to fight fatigue. It calms thirst more effectively than any other type of drink.
- It is an **excellent natural solution to treat hypertension**. In combination with garlic, lemons have demonstrated to be an effective natural remedy to cure hypertension. You can make a preparation of lemon juice combined with three crushed garlic cloves and one chopped onion plus 1 quart of low fat milk or soy milk. Boil all these

ingredients and drink this healthy potion to get the results.
- It helps **to lower your cholesterol naturally** thanks to the strength of pectin contained in this fruit.
- Drinking natural lemon juice also helps **to improve liver functions** since it regulates blood carbohydrate levels which influence blood oxygen levels. To relieve liver problems naturally you can drink a glass of hot water with lemon juice 1 hour prior to breakfast on a daily basis to get the benefits.
- It is great **to release the pain cause by a corn**, you can put a slice of lemon overnight over the affected area during the night to feel relieve.
- **To treat asthma** you can drink a teaspoon of lemon 1 hour prior to meals.

PAPAYA: the beneficial powers of eating papaya are countless. On top of being one of the most delicious fruits you can include in your healthy daily menu, **papayas are full of great vitamins and key nutrients**. They are a marvelous source of dietary fiber, vitamin A, vitamin C and vitamin E. They also hold some quantities of niacin, thiamine, folate, iron and calcium. Another great property of papayas is that they are **full of antioxidants nutrients like carotenes and flavonoids** and they contain high amounts of vitamin C and vitamin A. Another benefit of this delicious juicy fruit is that it is low in calories and low in sodium.

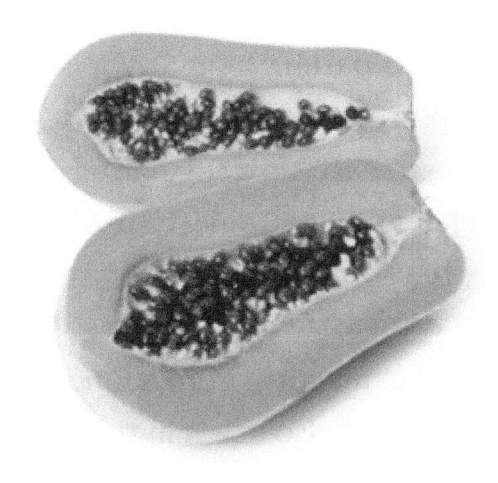

Here is a list of some of the best health powers of eating papaya:

- It helps to ease the pain from Rheumatoid arthritis and from osteoarthritis, it has powerful **natural anti-inflammatory properties** and make is it a great food for those who practice sports frequently.
- It is very **good to prevent diseases** like atherosclerosis and to prevent heart attacks.
- **It boosts the strength of your immune system naturally.** It is a good idea to eat papaya after an antibiotic treatment since its consumption helps to

replenish the bacterial balance that has been disrupted due to the antibiotics inside your system.
- Eating papaya after meals is a very healthy practice **to improve your digestive system functions** and **to prevent constipation**. It also avoids bloating and indigestion problems.
- Consuming papaya on a regular basis also **helps to cleanse the colon** naturally **to prevent colon cancer** and it is great for losing weight fast.
- It promotes the recovery muscle tissue.
- Papaya peel can be used on wounds so they heal faster or you can also use it in the form of papaya ointment to nourish skin and to moisturize
- It **promotes the good functioning of the cardiovascular system**.
- It is a great natural revitalizer that provides energy to your body and it can also be taken in the form of natural supplements.

PINEAPPLE: originally from South America this very juicy and sweet delicious fruit has many healthy powers. Although being a sweet fruit it is very low in calories (approx. 50 calories per 100 g) and **it has a high amount of soluble and insoluble dietary fiber** which makes it ideal for those wanting to lose weight. Here is a list of the best health powers of pineapples:

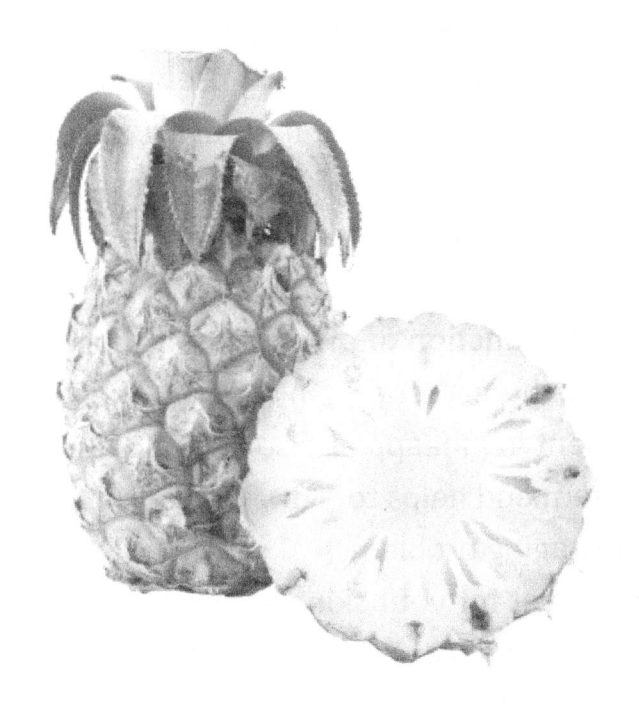

- Consuming pineapples **has anti-inflammatory properties** and they contain a powerful enzyme called **bromelain** that improves your digestive functions naturally. This enzyme helps to break down proteins and also has **anti-cancer and anti-clotting benefits**.

- To fight arthritis it is advisable to consume pineapple frequently according to studies and this also **helps with indigestion problems**
- Pineapples are a great natural source of antioxidants and vitamin C to promote collagen synthesis in your system. By maintaining a healthy collagen structure your body is able **to maintain the proper function of blood vessels**, bones, the skin and all human organs in general. The vitamin C present in pineapples also **boosts your immune system** and helps to fight free radicals preventing early aging problems.
- It is **great for your skin** and for your vision since it contains high amounts of vitamin A and beta-carotene levels.
- Pineapples are rich in manganese, copper and potassium making them and ideal fruit to eat **to control healthy blood pressure** and to maintain a healthy heart rate.
- Eating pineapples will help you **to maintain the health of your gums** in optimal conditions by strengthening them naturally
- Eating this juicy delicious fruit also **helps to reduce the risk of macular degeneration or vision loss** caused by the destruction of the retina. By including this healthy superfood into your diet you can reduce the risk of having this problem by as much

as 35% due to the beta-carotene contained inside pineapples.

MANGO: this mostly a tropical fruit but it is also a seasonable delicious fruit that you can get mainly during the summer time. This yummy fruit has several health powers; here is a list of all the benefits you can get from mangoes:

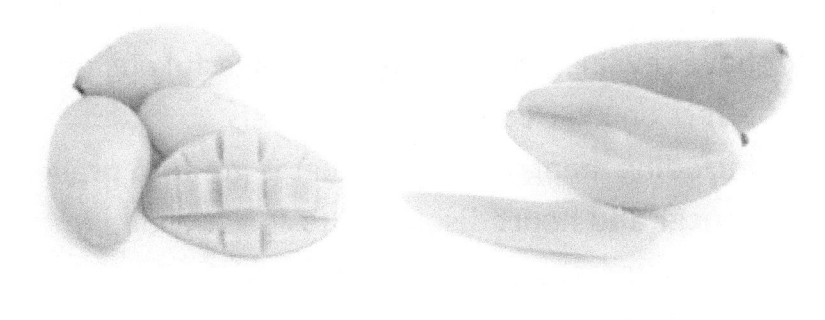

- Mangoes are a great source of **vitamin E** and it is a great food **to increase your sex drive** and it is among one of the best aphrodisiac foods you can take.
- Eating mangoes is very beneficial to improve your digestion; they contain enzymes that solve indigestion issues naturally and effectively.
- One very useful power of mangoes is **to treat acne**. It helps to clean pores that cause acne. The way to

use mango for this purpose is to slice it into thin pieces and put those slices on your face affected area for about 15 minutes approximately and then clean your face with warm water.
- Due to its high amounts of soluble dietary fiber, **vitamin C and Pectin**, mangoes are great to lower bad cholesterol levels naturally.
- By consuming mangoes frequently **you improve your memory**. The Glutamine acid contained in mangoes has been tested in different studies that have revealed a boosting and powerful positive effect on kid's concentration levels.
- Including mangoes in your diet is great **to prevent cancer and heart diseases**. It is a good idea to eat mangoes frequently to profit from its high amounts of **anti-cancer antioxidants**.
- Mangoes are also full of iron and are a great natural alternative for people with anemia. **Mangoes are great for pregnant women** and for women after menopause to increase the levels of energy naturally.
- It is also great to fight diabetes. The best way to consume mangoes for this purpose is to drink a glass of warm water with mango leaves. You should leave the leaves inside the water during the night and drink this healthy portion first thing in the morning on a regular basis to get all the benefits.

- It can also be taken in the form of natural supplements to lose weight faster and to boost metabolism naturally.

AVOCADOS: avocados are not only delicious but they also have anti-cancer properties. They are also a great natural food to include in a healthy low cholesterol diet. Avocados are among the richer sources of nutrients and vitamins you can find in nature. They are a great source of potassium, dietary fiber, vitamin B6, vitamin C, **vitamin K**, folic acid and copper and it is no surprise why some consider avocados the healthiest fruit on earth. Here is a list of some of the health powers of avocados:

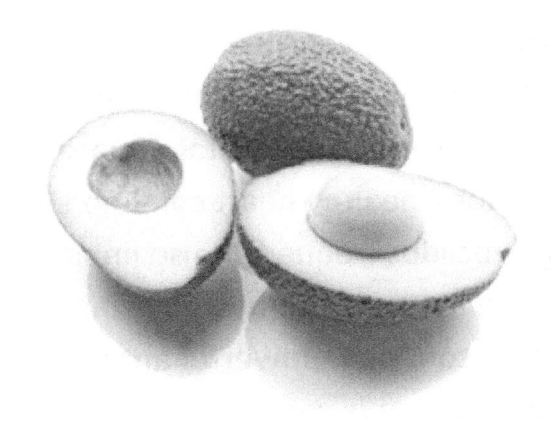

- Eating avocados frequently is great to prevent the appearance of certain types of cancer like breast cancer and prostate cancer. They contain monounsaturated fatty acids and oleic acid which have shown **positive health effects against breast cancer** in recent studies. According to some studies a substance contained in avocados can destroy cancer cells naturally.
- Eating avocados is very beneficial to lower bad cholesterol levels naturally. According to some studies people who included avocados in their diets showed notable health improvements and lower cholesterol levels.
- It helps **to control blood pressure** naturally due the high amounts of potassium it contains. It is a great food to include in your menu to prevent circulatory related diseases like high blood pressure and heart attacks. **Avocados also contain folate**, an essential nutrient for a healthy heart condition.
- Eating avocados frequently also improves your body's ability to absorb nutrients more effectively.
- **Avocados contain a powerful antioxidant called Glutathione** that is very beneficial to prevent premature aging, to prevent cancer and to prevent heart disease naturally and effectively.
- **When you eat avocados your eye´s health improves notably**. This fruit has amazing powerful

effects on your eyes due to the high amounts of carotenoid lutein they contain. **Lutein** protects against cataracts and macular degeneration.

You can consume this delicious superfood with salads, with tuna, with fish, in the form of juice or as a great complement of many healthy dishes.

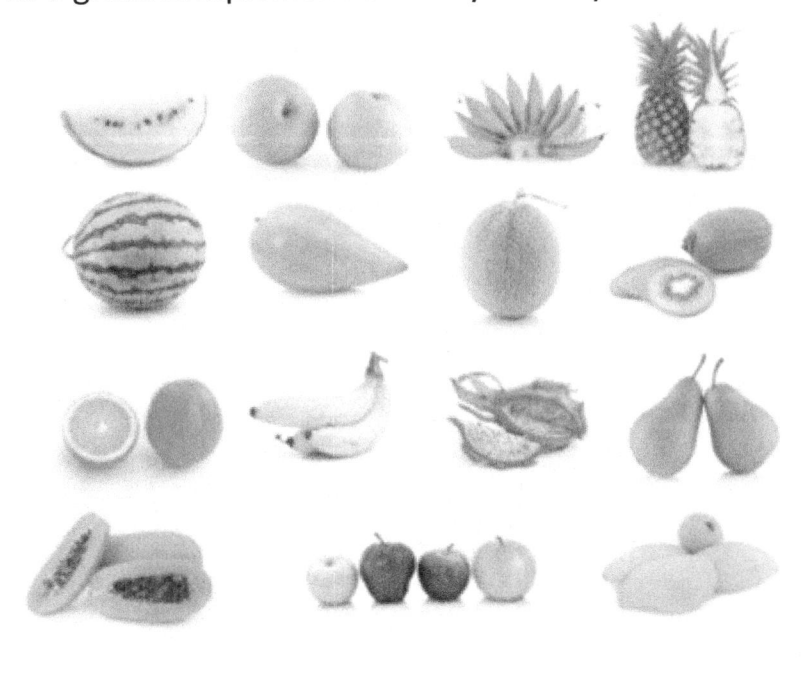

POMEGRANATE: it is been considered as one of the top fruits in terms of healthy beneficial powers.

Consuming this fruit has shown to be a very powerful natural solution to fight Alzheimer´s disease, coronary disease, heart problems and **to prevent various types of cancers**. It has plenty of antioxidants that are beneficial for your health; here is a list of some of the health powers that this fruit has to offer:

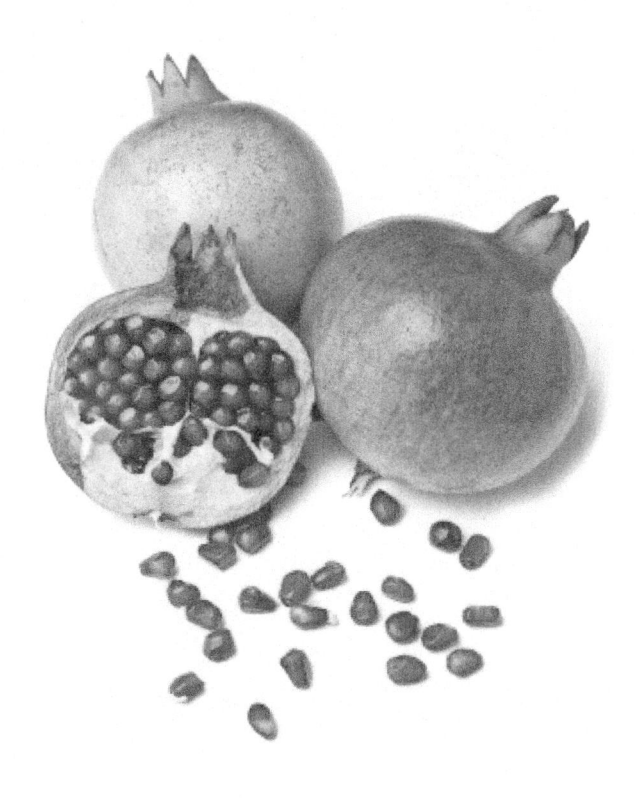

- This fruit is full of antioxidants that help **to boost your immune system** naturally
- According to some recent studies including pomegranate juice in your diet may **reduce the risk of many types of cancers** and also it may be beneficial to fight prostate cancer naturally and effectively.
- Consuming pomegranate in the form of juice is also beneficial for your skin health
- It reduces the risk of developing Alzheimer's disease
- According to some studies including this powerful fruit in your diet can **help to diminish the risk of the appearance of certain diseases** like atherosclerosis, diabetes and osteoarthritis. These illnesses are caused by the hardening and thickening of arterial walls and drinking pomegranate juice may help in reducing those risks naturally.
- Different studies also have shown the powers of pomegranate to **diminish the risk of having heart attacks** and its ability to promote healthy blood circulation. It prevents the formation of arteries clots and keeps your cholesterol levels healthy.
- Taken in the form of natural supplements pomegranates has also demonstrated to be very beneficial in promoting **Nitric Oxide** production

inside the body **to improve circulation** and **to improve male sexual performance.**

ONIONS: this vegetable is a superfood full of nutritional benefits and vitamins. Onions contain dietary fiber (1.5 grams approx.), vitamin C, vitamin B6, chromium, biotin and calcium. They also are **a good source of vitamin B1**, folic acid and vitamin B1. The substance that causes your eyes to get irritated when you chop the onions is called **alliianase**, the same substance is present in garlic. They also are **provided with healthy antioxidants like flavonoids** that have healthy benefits like preventing tumors and immune system enhancing properties. Another key element present in onions is **sulfur**, a substance **very beneficial for your liver health**.

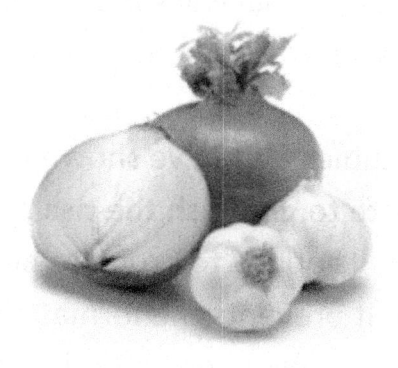

- Eating onions helps you **to lower your bad cholesterol levels** naturally thanks to a substance called quercitin. This substance also **improves blood circulation** by making your blood thinner. This characteristic makes onions part of the best aphrodisiac foods since it improves circulation to your genital parts.
- Eating onions helps **to prevent artery clot formation**
- It helps to prevent asthma, chronic bronchitis, diabetes, fever and atherosclerosis.
- It has **anti-cancer powers** and prevents the appearance of stomach cancer.
- Sulfur compounds inside onions also make them an excellent choice to detoxify your body naturally. By eating onions on a regular basis your system is able to get rid of mercury, lead and cadmium residues naturally and effectively.
- Onions have powerful anti-cancer benefits since eating them can reduce the damage caused by free radicals and diminishing the harm caused to cells and DNA
- It can help **to eliminate tumor cells** and stop the growth of tumors according to some studies. For this purpose it can be consumed in the form of onion extract to get all the benefits.

- By including onions in your healthy menus you are able **to control sugar levels in your blood** naturally. In fact eating onions can help to lower blood sugar levels very effectively and it is an excellent natural alternative to replace prescription drugs.
- Consuming onions is also a great natural alternative **to treat asthma** since they relax bronchial muscles naturally
- Another great benefit of onions is that they have **powerful antibacterial properties** and can get rid of pathogens like E. coli and salmonella naturally and effectively.

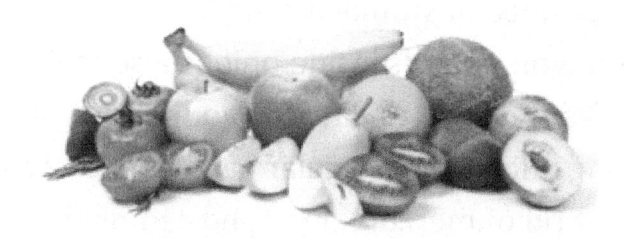

CARROTS: carrots have a delicious and crispy texture that makes it an ideal vegetable to eat at any time as a healthy snack or to mix it with salads or other great dishes. This very popular vegetable has **great amounts of nutrients and vitamins** that make it **an ideal choice to include it in your healthy menus to feel and look better.** They are an excellent source of dietary fiber, thiamine, biotin, and vitamins like vitamin B1, vitamin B2, vitamin B6 and vitamin K. The following is a list of some of the best health powers you get when you eat carrots:

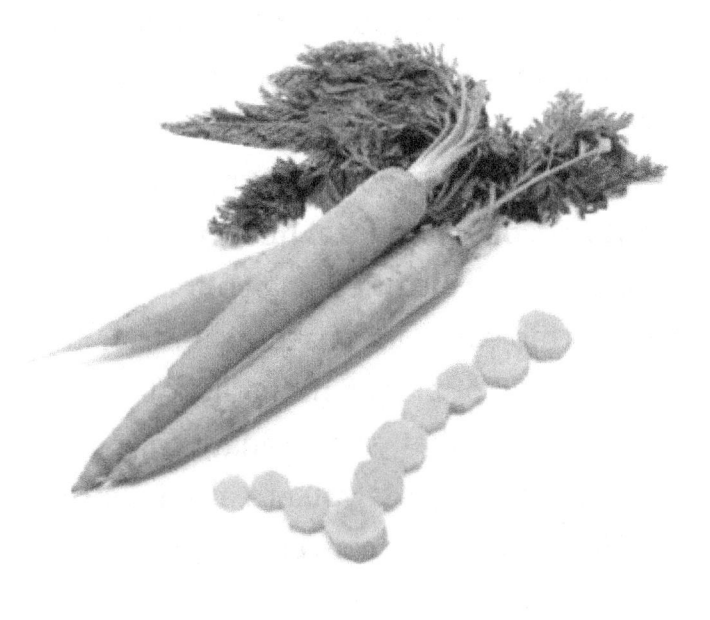

- Eating carrots has **anti-aging powers**. This wonderful and delicious sweet vegetable contains beta-carotene, **a powerful antioxidant** that contributes to maintain the body's health against free radicals. When you eat carrots on a regular basis your body cells benefit by **slowing down the aging process**.
- This great vegetable has also powerful body detoxifying properties and cleansing powers that are great **to detox your liver naturally** and

effectively. By eating carrots you also improve your skin conditions and you get rid of acne caused by toxins inside your system. It has powerful nutrients and vitamin A that **nourishes your skin** making it look younger and healthier.

- Including carrots in your daily menu is great **to maintain a proper dental health**. When you eat carrots you are also cleaning your teeth because this vegetable acts as a natural abrasive that helps you to get rid of plaque naturally. Also carrots are full of minerals that give strength to your teeth.
- When you eat carrots you are also **lowering the risk of different types of cancers** like colon cancer, breast cancer and lung cancer. One of the key components that make this yummy vegetable so **anti-cancer** friendly is a substance called falcarinol, a natural compound that also transforms this vegetable in a good resource to fight fungal diseases. This ingredient makes carrots an excellent natural superfood to prevent the appearance of cancer according to recent studies.
- **Eating carrots is excellent for improving vision**. It provides essential vitamin A to the retina of the eye, the absence of vitamin A causes night blindness. Carrots have also high amounts of **beta-carotene** that is very beneficial for your eyes health and to prevent macular degeneration. Eating foods

with high amounts of beta-carotene **helps to reduce the risk of developing cataracts** and macular degeneration.
- Carrots contain carotenoids that are an excellent natural compound to prevent heart disease.
- Eating carrots frequently also helps **to reduce bad cholesterol levels** and it is a great natural ingredient to include in every low cholesterol diet.

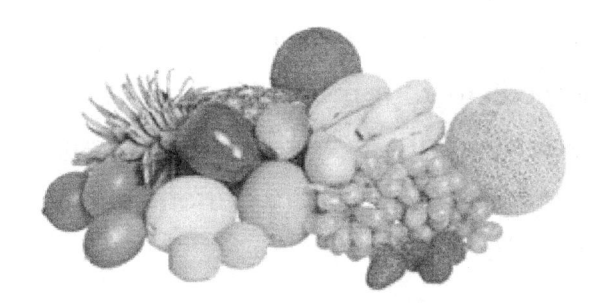

BROCCOLI: this vegetable really is an amazing superfood that has many health benefits. Here is a list of the benefits your get when you include this very healthy vegetable into your diet:

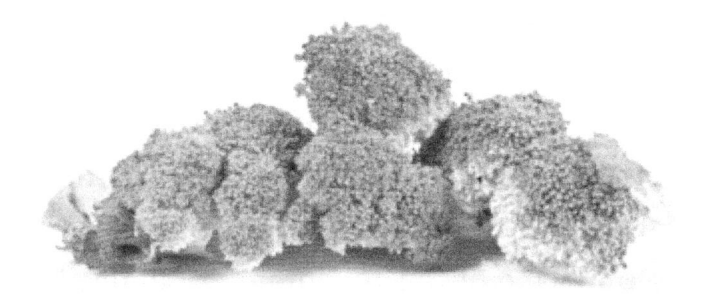

- It is very beneficial **to control blood pressure naturally** thanks of being rich in nutrients like magnesium, calcium and potassium.
- Eating broccoli is great for your bones health since it has generous amounts of calcium and vitamin K; these two components also help **to avoid the presence of osteoporosis**.
- Due to its richness in potassium, the inclusion of broccoli in your menu can help **to promote a healthy nervous system** and a healthy brain function. It is also very beneficial to boost muscle growth.
- Including broccoli in your diet **helps to prevent cancer**. This vegetable has a powerful anti-cancer component called **glucoraphanin** that when consumed your system transforms it into the anti-cancer substance sulforaphane.
- Broccoli is an **excellent natural food with high amounts of dietary fiber** that makes it ideal for a healthy weight loss diet. This dietary fiber inside this vegetable helps **to promote healthy bowel movements**, to improve digestion. Eating broccoli also **helps to control the levels of sugar in your blood**. One of the advantages of eating broccoli for

fast weight loss is that one cup of this vegetable has as much dietary fiber as a cup of rice or corn with fewer calories.

- Eating broccoli improves your heart's health. This wonderful vegetable contains carotenoid lutein that on top of preventing heart disease **it also prevents the thickening of your arteries**. You also reduce the risk of having a stroke when you eat broccoli a regular basis since its **vitamin B6** improves circulation and **diminishes the risk of developing atherosclerosis**.
- When you eat broccoli **your immune system is improved naturally**. Broccoli is rich in beta-carotene, zinc and selenium.
- Eating broccoli improve liver function notably thanks to its powerful antioxidants
- Carotenoid lutein present in broccoli **promotes your eyes health**. This ingredient is beneficial to prevent age-related macular degeneration effectively and also to prevent the appearance of cataracts. Broccoli is also an excellent source of **vitamin A**, this vitamin is essential to preserve the ability of night vision and **to strengthen the retina**. You can also get the benefits of broccoli in the form of <u>natural supplements</u>.
- **Eating broccoli helps your skin to recover from sun damage naturally**. It contains a powerful natural

ingredient called glucoraphanin that helps to the natural repair of damaged skin also preventing skin cancer.

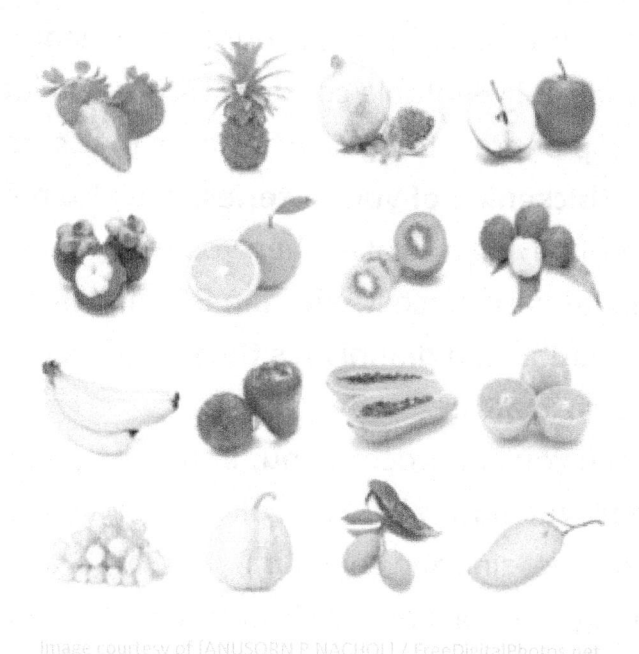

Image courtesy of [ANUSORN P NACHOL] / FreeDigitalPhotos.net

SPINACH: this vegetable should be on the top of your list if you want to give your body all the benefits and health powers it contains. Here is a list of the best benefits you get when you consume this healthy vegetable:

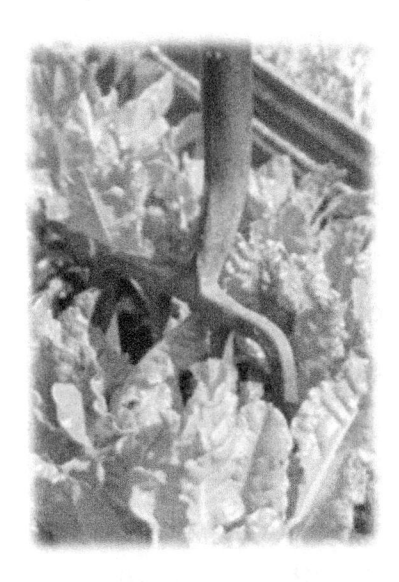

- Eating spinaches has great **anti-inflammatory benefits**. This healthy vegetable contains high amounts of two powerful ingredients, **violaxanthin** and **neoxanthin** that help **to control inflammation naturally**.
- This vegetable is great **to control healthy blood pressure** since it contains peptides that help to regulate blood pressure naturally.
- Spinach is **full of antioxidants** like vitamin C, vitamin E, beta-carotene, zinc, manganese and selenium. All this powerful ingredients help to fight atherosclerosis, high blood pressure and osteoporosis.

- Flavonoids present in spinach make them a great natural food for **anti-cancer purposes**. This phytonutrient has **powerful anti-cancer benefits** and it is contained in high amounts inside spinach. This ingredient has been shown to control and detain the proliferation of cancer cells in humans.
- Eating spinach is very beneficial **to improve vision** since it has two key components called lutein and zeaxanthin that protect your eyes against cataracts and all age-related eye diseases.
- It is **good for your skin**. Spinach is full of **vitamin A** that gives your skin a healthier and younger look by providing natural moisture and preventing the appearance of psoriasis, acne, wrinkles and different types of skin illnesses.
- When you eat spinach **your bones are fortified** thanks to the high amount of **vitamin K** they contain.
- Vitamin K present in spinach also helps your body **to fight atherosclerosis and cardiovascular diseases**. Vitamin K in spinach also promotes a healthy nervous system.

SANTOL: This powerful and exotic rare delicious fruit is found in abundant quantities in the Philippines and in Thailand. This exotic fruit is usually consumed raw and without peeling but it is also used to make marmalade and it can be found in some supermarkets in jars in the form of marmalade or contained in glass jars. It is not too common to find this exotic fruit also known as "sandorica" but it has some great properties and health benefits.

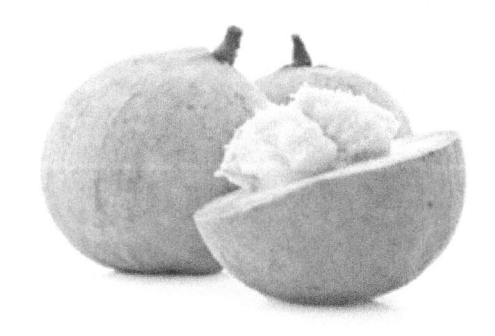

Here are some of the uses of the Santol Fruit:

- It **helps to cure fever** naturally when the leaves are placed on the body skin, the leaves can be cooked to obtain a healing natural potion to bath the ill person.
- It can also be used **to cure itching skin**.
- It can be used to cure diarrhea when its root is crushed and blended with vinegar and water and can be drunk as a natural remedy.

- The root can also be consumed **to energize the body** naturally.

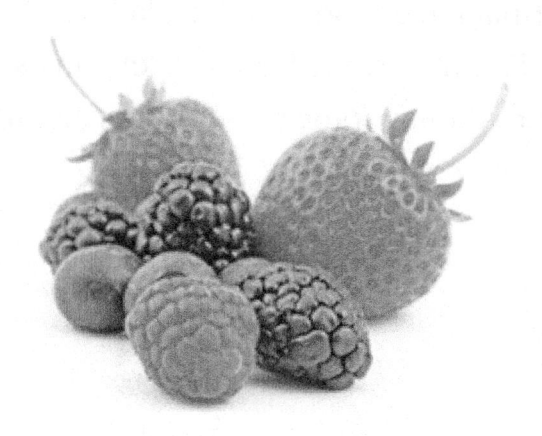

TOMATOES: tomatoes are considered both a fruit and a vegetable and they truly have very beneficial health powers. Eating tomatoes is good to control hypertension; it is good for skin problems, for diabetes, to improve eye health and to cure urinary tract infections among many other benefits. This great natural superfood is ideal to add not only flavor to your meals but also **to improve your health notably**. It is **full of powerful and effective antioxidants** that help to prevent many types of cancers and also full of vitamins and nutrients that empower your entire overall health condition. Here is a description of the best health powers you can get from eating tomatoes on a regular basis:

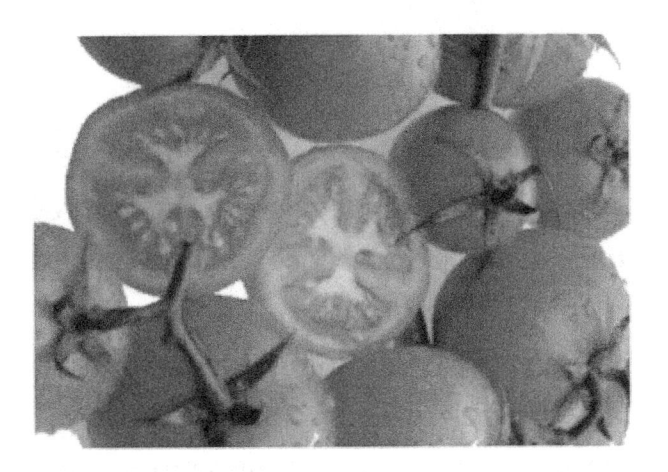

- Consuming tomatoes frequently **helps to improve vision naturally** and effectively. This vegetable has high amounts of vitamin A preventing macular degeneration.
- It is one of the best natural superfoods you can eat to give your body all the vitamins it needs. Just one tomato alone has approximately 40% of the daily vitamin C your body needs. This natural antioxidant is a strong natural anti-cancer agent that fights against free radicals that intoxicate your system. Another key nutrient found in tomatoes is potassium; this is great **for improving your nervous system health**. Tomatoes also have iron and **vitamin A** to help you keep a healthy circulatory system and to prevent blood clots.

- Consuming tomatoes is very beneficial **to lower high blood pressure**
- It is great to avoid urinary tract infections
- When you eat tomatoes frequently you **reduce the chances of the appearance of gallstones**, it helps to dissolve them naturally
- It improves the health of your skin naturally and it is a great anti-aging food
- Tomatoes have two key components that are very beneficial for those looking to quit smoking. **Coumaric acid** and **chlorogenic acid** help to fight against the effects of nitrosamines which are one of the main components found in cigarettes.
- It is very recommendable to eat tomatoes to maintain a healthy digestive system **to prevent constipation and diarrhea**. This food acts as a natural detoxifying agent inside your system **cleansing your body from toxins.**
- According to some studies eating tomatoes is very beneficial to relieve diabetes symptoms.
- An ingredient found in tomatoes called lycopene **protects your body against cardiovascular diseases**. Also frequent consumption of tomatoes helps to reduce bad cholesterol levels and triglycerides in your blood.
- This red and delicious vegetable is packed with healthy and beneficial antioxidants that **protect**

your body against many types of cancers. A very effective substance inside this vegetable called lycopene is especially powerful to **prevent certain types of cancers** like cervical cancer, stomach cancer, prostate cancer, pharynx cancer and rectum cancer among others. It is also a great natural food to consume for women who want **to prevent the appearance of breast cancer** according to studies performed in the Harvard School of Public Health.

So enjoy this yummy vegetable whenever you can and include it in your healthy menus and salads as often as you can to get all the powers this magical superfood has to offer.

Maca Root: this is one of the most powerful "superfoods" that can be found in nature.

Maca is considered one of the most powerful

"superfoods" that we can consume to improve the health of our body. Many people believe that these small roots possess amazing **magical powers**, but scientific analysis done on the properties of this root show is really an amazing resource of good nutrition. Maca root contains many nutrients that feed the brain, repair hormonal irregularities naturally and improves sexual at the same time.

Maca root is a really powerful natural food full of nutrients; it contains lots of very beneficial vitamins, several essential minerals, plant sterols, amino acids and healthy fats. This is a great powerful food for athletes and for those seeking to combat stress or to increase stamina.

Consuming maca may affect men and women differently. Men usually use it to enhance fertility and sexual performance. Both men and women found that it can significantly increase libido and sex drive, it also increases energy, stamina and the sense wellbeing. For women it is great to help relieve the symptoms of PMS and menopause.

What are the origins of this amazing root?

It is grown in the highlands of Peru at altitudes of 7,000 to 12,000 feet, and beyond, it is the plant that grows at higher altitudes in the entire planet. This plant has been used by native Peruvians since the mid-15th century. Since this plant grew spontaneously in the wild, it quickly became a staple of the daily diet of the natives, and eaten raw or cooked.

Maca is a radish root vegetable and is related to the potato family, is considered a sacred tuber and is has a spherical shape. The root is between three and six inches in diameter and approximately of the same length. There are four recognized types of Maca, based on the color of the root, which vary from creamy yellow to pale pink to deep purple or even dark.

Maca root is known as a natural restorative, which means it increases the body's ability to defend itself against physical and mental weakening, and thus protects us from diseases. This is achieved by providing support to the adrenal and pituitary gland health, which supports the proper functioning of the endocrine gland.

Nutritional Content of Maca:

Maca root is a super nutritional root, with close to sixty different phytonutrients! These phytochemicals combined make this vegetable an amazing food full of vitamins and this is why it is considered to be one of the most powerful medicinal plants of the earth.

Maca contains significant amounts of amino acids, carbohydrates and minerals like calcium, phosphorus, zinc, magnesium, iron, and vitamins B1, B2, B12, C and E.

Unlike herbs that can have negative effects when used improperly, maca has no known contraindications or toxicity. However, occasionally some people experience side effects when they start taking it, these symptoms could be signs of the detoxifying effects of the plant.

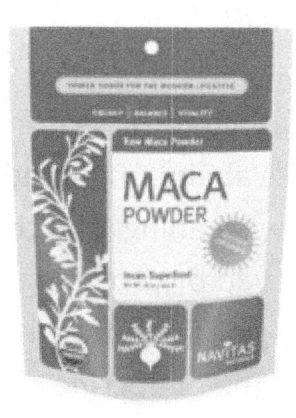

Ways to use Maca as Food:

The most common way to use this root as a food is in the form of <u>maca powder</u>. Maca powder is a very powerful food, and with just a little sprinkle on food this transforms any food into super healthy nourishment. Maca powder has an earthy flavor that is slightly nutty, with a hint of caramel. It's easy to mix in milk shakes or mixed with flour for dessert recipes. It can be also used in the form of [natural supplements](#) to increase sexual potency for men.

You can also consume maca powder by adding it to healthy vegetables soups to increase their healing powers and health properties. Another option is to add it to natural drinks like herbal tea or green tea to detoxify your system. It should be used in small quantities so you get all the benefits.

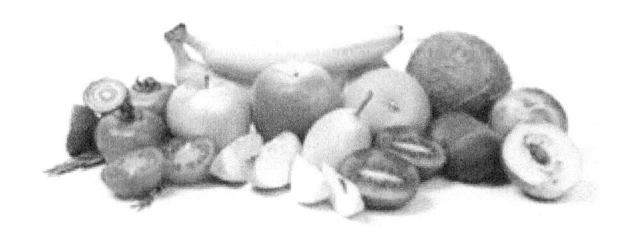

GARLIC: garlic is not only an amazing natural food that gives great taste to our dishes but it also has marvelous healing powers and it is **a great healthy food** to include in our menus **to prevent many diseases**. Among the many benefits of eating garlic are its anti-cancer powers, **heart**

disease prevention and even a natural cure for impotence. Here is a list of the best health powers you can benefit from when you make garlic a part of your healthy menus:

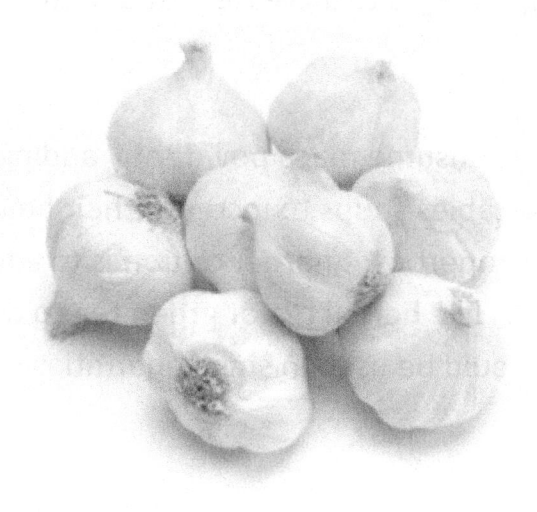

Image courtesy of [SUAT EMAN] / FreeDigitalPhotos.net

- Garlic is a great natural food that can **cure impotence** problems and it is considered one of the most powerful aphrodisiac foods. Eating this healthy food keeps arteries and veins in good condition and **improves circulation to your genital areas**. It stimulates the production of an enzyme called **Nitric Oxide** naturally to boost erections. Nitric Oxide makes the blood vessels to dilate and also make the blood flow stronger especially to your genital areas.

- Eating garlic is great **to prevent heart disease**. It is very beneficial to lower bad cholesterol levels and **to prevent blood clots**. When you eat garlic you also **raise your good cholesterol levels naturally**, this diminishes the risk of the formation of plaque in the arteries. You can eat two cloves a day to help your body to maintain optimal cholesterol levels and **prevent heart disease or a stroke**.
- Including garlic in your daily menus is great **to boost your immune system** and to prevent many types of cancers. It reduces the risk of cancerous cells formation and at the same type it **reduces the risk of developing cancer tumors**. Compounds inside garlic can even **reduce the size of a tumor**. Consuming garlic is great **to prevent breast cancer and prostate cancer**. Two ingredients inside garlic make this natural superfood very powerful against cancer, these ingredients are: **s-allycystein and diallye disulphide**. These two compounds are released when garlic is crushed. Another sulfur components in garlic are the ones called **ajoenes** that have strong anti-tumor powers.
- Garlic is excellent to treat cold naturally. You can eat some cloves of garlic to get rid of colds without the use of drugs. **Your immune system turns**

stronger when you eat garlic since it contains powerful antioxidants that give your immune system a natural boost.

- By eating garlic you **control your blood pressure naturally**. Your blood gets thinner when you eat garlic. A substance called ajoene inside garlic is responsible for this power of making your blood thinner and thus improving circulation. **Avoid hypertension problems** by including this healthy superfood in your daily diet.
- Consuming garlic is an excellent choice for women who are pregnant. It reduces the risk of malformations in the baby according to some studies and also helps babies to grow healthier. It also is very beneficial **to improve memory**. Garlic is also great to detox your body naturally due to its high levels of antioxidants. Eat at least 6 cloves a day while detoxifying your body naturally to get all the benefits of the sulfur it contains. You can eat it raw or cooked.
- Garlic has strong **anti-bacterial properties** that help to fight infection naturally and effectively. In fact Louis Pasteur made the discovery that bacterial cells died when they were exposed to garlic. It can be used as a natural anti-biotic agent and it also has **anti-viral powers**. When you are having problems

with intestinal parasites it is a good idea to consume garlic **to get rid of viruses and infections**.

Just two cloves of raw garlic every day will really keep doctors away. You can also take them in the form of natural supplements to get all the benefits.

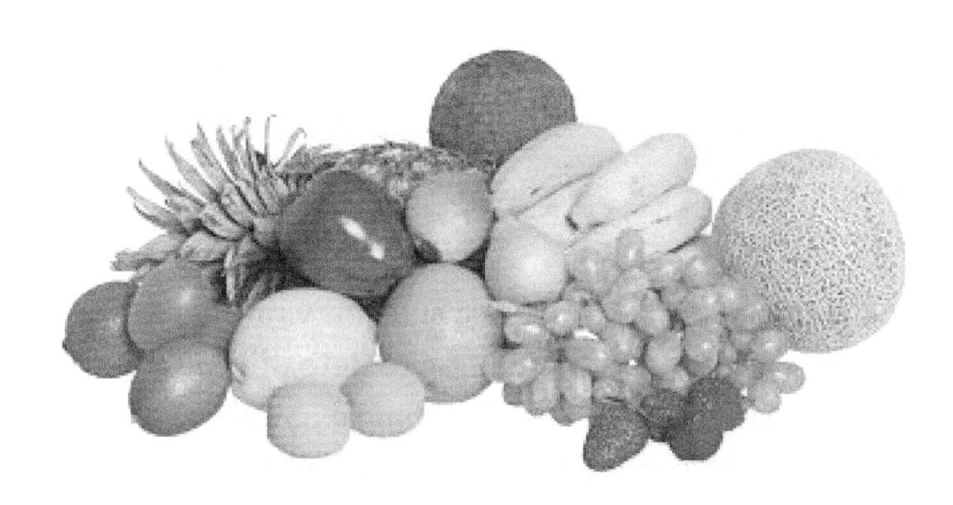

GINGER: this natural root is considered more of a spice than a fruit or a vegetable but it has **incredible health powers** that can be obtained when used for different food preparations. Ginger is a perennial plant that has its origins in China. It can be taken in the form of natural supplements or it can be added to different healthy recipes. This plant is known for its strong spicy aroma due to its high concentration of natural essential oils. The part of the plant that is commercialized is the rhizoid and can be eaten. You can also find it in the form of powder and in the form of healthy ginger organic tonic.

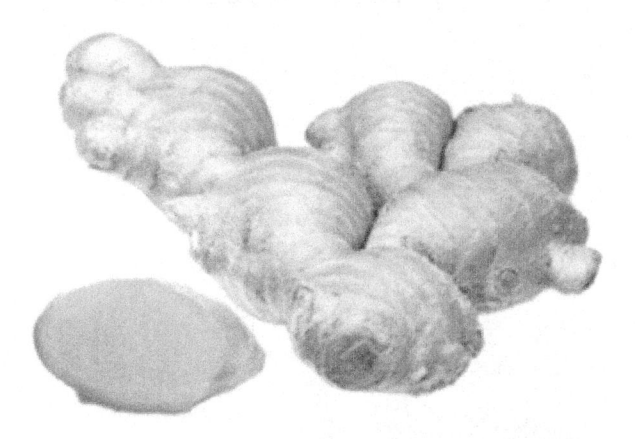

- Ginger is full of anti-toxic and anti-viral agents and it is a great natural solution **to detoxify your body effectively**. It also has anti-fungal powers and eating this root can help to fight common cold symptoms.
- Ginger has powerful anti-inflammatory properties and it is great to treat arthritis and osteoarthritis.
- Consuming ginger help your digestive system to function properly due to the special enzymes it contains. These enzymes catalyze the proteins in the foods you consume making your digestion process much smoother and easier. It is great **to**

cure gastrointestinal problems and indigestion naturally.
- Including ginger in your diet and your recipes can help to lower bad cholesterol levels naturally and also **prevent the formation of blood clots** thus preventing heart disease problems.
- Ginger stimulates the secretion of mucus inside your stomach preventing the appearance of ulcers.
- It also can help to relieve your stomach from bloating and gas problems.
- Consuming ginger is also great **to fight cough and to sooth sore throat** problems.
- Consuming ginger can cure the feelings of nausea, morning sickness and it is an excellent natural solution to cure side effects caused by chemotherapy.
- Ginger also has antihistamine powers to **help you treat allergy problems naturally**.
- Ginger can be used to treat diarrhea and to cure upset stomach problems naturally.
- Ginger also **promotes healthy circulation** and relaxes blood vessels thus improving blood flow thought the entire body; this is why it is also considered to be among the best aphrodisiac foods.

Ginger can be used to cook many spicy healthy recipes and it is a great idea to include it in your menus to get all the **healthy powers** it has to offer so you can start looking and feeling much better now. Ginger root can also be taken in the form of natural supplements.

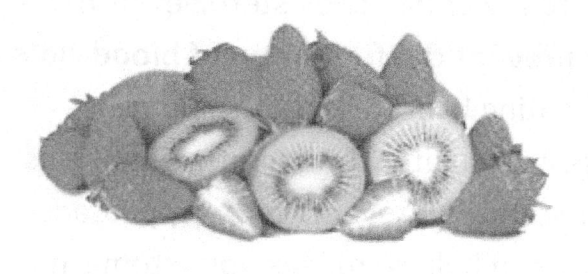

KIWI: this funny named fruit can really be considered a **superfood** due to its powerful health benefits. Kiwi has a reputation of being one of the most nutritious fruits on earth. It is the fruit with the highest amount of folate and vitamin K. Here is a list of the most important health powers you get from consuming this delicious fruit:

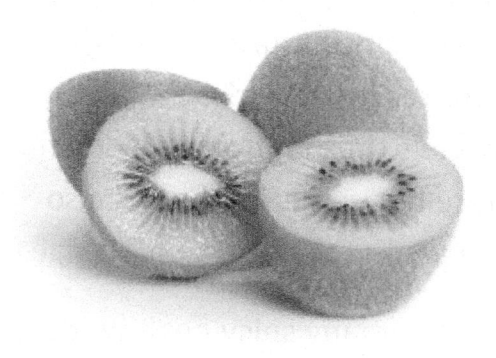

- Consuming kiwi often will help you **to strengthen your bones** due to the high amounts of vitamin K found inside this yummy fruit. Vitamin K is an essential healthy nutrient that strengthens bone metabolism naturally. When there is an insufficiency of vitamin K in the body the risks of developing osteoporosis are higher.
- Eating kiwis on a regular basis help **to improve your bowel movements** naturally and help **to prevent constipation problems** thanks to the high amounts of dietary fiber it has.
- Kiwi is one of the fruits with the highest amounts of vitamin C and this makes this delicious fruit one of the best superfoods **to prevent asthma** thanks to its anti-inflammatory powers.
- Kiwi contains calcium and also **vitamin K**; these two nutrients make kiwi an excellent **healthy blood flow** promoter **to avoid blood clotting problems**.
- When you eat kiwis you also **avoid muscle soreness**. It is an excellent natural food to soothe muscle soreness, muscle tension, muscle cramps and muscle fatigue. The **Magnesium** contained inside the kiwi fruit is responsible for these **natural muscle healing properties**. Magnesium relaxes your

muscles and relaxes your nerves naturally and effectively.

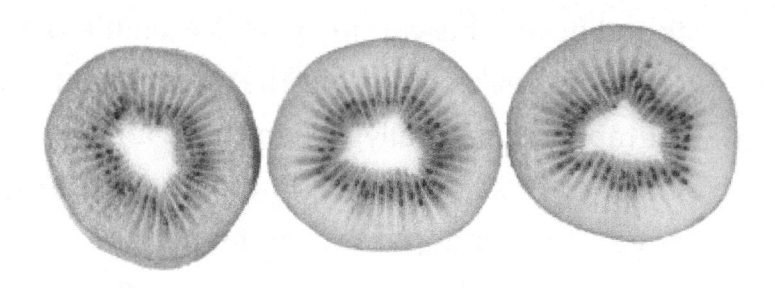

- Eating kiwi also **helps to prevent anemia** thanks to the folate it contains. Anemia is caused in part when there is vitamin B12 and folate deficiency.
- Eating kiwi helps as a **natural energy booster** thanks to the **potassium** it contains.
- When you eat kiwis your body produces more melanin thanks to key amino acids like **L-phenylalanine** and copper present in this wonderful and healthy fruit. This is very beneficial to maintain the color of your hair, a **healthy skin and healthy eyes**.

- Eating kiwi fruit is also beneficial **to regulate blood sugar levels** naturally thanks to the Manganese it contains.
- When you include kiwis in your daily diet you are also **helping your skin** to **reduce wrinkles** because kiwis are rich in **vitamin E** that **improve your skin** look and texture naturally.

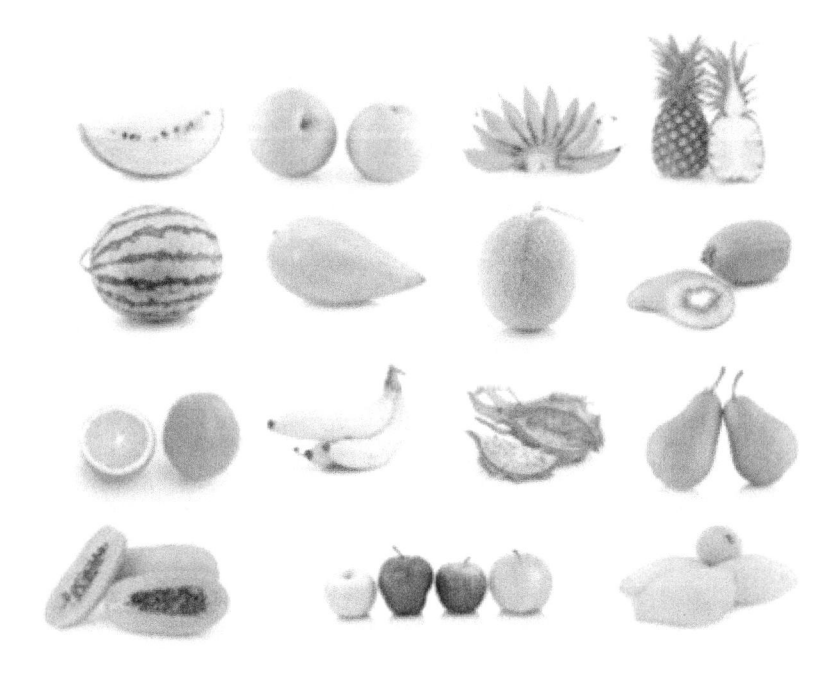

HERE IS A VERY HELPFUL CHART THAT ILLUSTRATES SOME OF THE BEST BENEFITS OF SOME OF THE MOST POWERFUL FRUITS AND VEGETABLES

FRUIT OR VEGETABLE	HEALTH POWER	HEALTH POWER	HEALTH POWER	HEALTH POWER	HEALTH POWER
APPLES	PROTECTS YOUR HEART	PREVENTS CONSTIPATION	STOPS DIARRHEA	IMPROVES LUNG CAPACITY	CUSSHIONS JOINTS
APRICOTS	FIGHTS CANCER	CONTROLS BLOOD PRESSURE	PROMOTES HEALTHY EYES	PROTECTS AGAINS ALZHEIMER´S	SLOWS AGING PROCESS
ARTICHOKES	HELPS DIGESTION	LOWERS CHOLESTEROL	PROTECTS YOUR HEART	STABILIZES BLOOD SUGAR	PROTECTS AGAINS LIVER DISEASE
AVOCADOS	FIGHTS DIABETES	LOWERS CHOLESTEROL	HELPS TO AVOID STROKES	CONTROLS BLOOD PRESSURE	SMOOTHES SKIN
BANANAS	PROTECTS YOUR HEART	QUIETS A COUGHT	STREGHTENS BONES	CONTROLS BLOOD PRESSURE	STOPS DIARRHEA
BEANS	PREVENTS CONSTIPATION	HELPS HEMORROIDS	LOWERS CHOLESTEROL	FIGHTS CANCER	STABILIZES BLOOD SUGAR
BEETS	CONTROLS BLOOD PRESSURE	FIGHTS CANCER	STREGHTENS BONES	PROTECTS YOUR HEART	AIDS WEIGHT LOSS
BLUEBERRIES	FIGHTS CANCER	PROTECTS YOUR HEART	STABLIZES BLOOD SUGAR	IMPROVES MEMORY	PRVENTS CONSTIPATION
BROCCOLI	STREGHTENS BONES	PROMOTES HEALTHY EYES	FIGHTS CANCER	PROTECTS YOUR HEART	CONTROLS BLOOD PRESSURE
CANTALOUPE	PROMOTES HEALTHY EYES	CONTROLS BLOOS PRESSURE	LOWERS CHOLESTEROL	FIGHTS CANCER	BOOSTS IMMUNE SYSTEM
CABBAGE	FIGHTS CANCER	PREVENTS CONSTIPATION	PROMOTES WEIGHT LOSS	PROTECTS YOUR HEART	HELPS HEMORROIDS

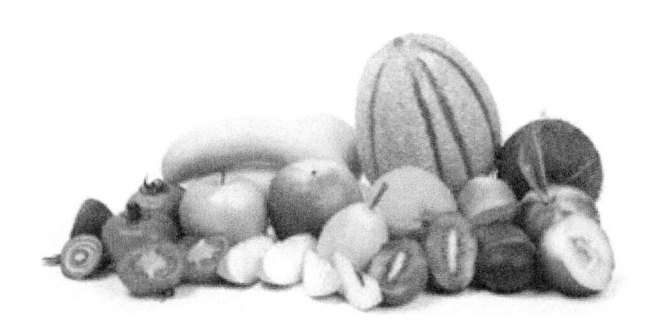

Image courtesy of [PIXOMAR] / FreeDigitalPhotos.net

List of the Amount of Fiber Contained in Fruits and Vegetables

TOTAL FIBER GRAMS (g)

Fresh & Dried Fruit	Serving Size	Amount of Fiber (g) Approx.
Apples with skin	1 medium	5.0
Apricot	3 medium	1.0
Apricots, dried	4 pieces	2.7
Banana	1 medium	3.5
Blueberries	1 cup	4.1
Cantaloupe, cubes	1 cup	1.5
Figs, dried	2 medium	3.5
Grapefruit	1/2 medium	3.0
Orange, navel	1 medium	3.3
Peach	1 medium	2.0
Peaches, dried	3 pieces	3.3
Pear	1 medium	5.2
Plum	1 medium	1.3
Raisins	1.5 oz box	1.5
Raspberries	1 cup	6.3
Strawberries	1 cup	4.3

Vegetables	Serving Size	Fiber (g)
Avocado (fruit)	1 medium	11.8
Beets, cooked	1 cup	2.8
Beet greens	1 cup	4.2
Bok choy, cooked	1 cup	2.8
Broccoli, cooked	1 cup	4.5
Brussels sprouts, cooked	1 cup	3.6
Cabbage, cooked	1 cup	4.2
Carrot	1 medium	2.6
Carrot, cooked	1 cup	5.2
Cauliflower, cooked	1 cup	3.4

Cole slaw	1 cup	4.0
Collard greens, cooked	1 cup	2.6
Corn, sweet	1 cup	4.6
Green beans	1 cup	4.0
Celery	1 stalk	1.1
Kale, cooked	1 cup	7.2
Onions, raw	1 cup	2.9
Peas, cooked	1 cup	8.8
Peppers, sweet	1 cup	2.6
Potato, baked w/ skin	1 medium	4.8
Spinach, cooked	1 cup	4.3
Summer squash, cooked	1 cup	2.5
Sweet potato, cooked	1 medium	4.9
Swiss chard, cooked	1 cup	3.7
Tomato	1 medium	1.0
Winter squash, cooked	1 cup	6.2
Zucchini, cooked	1 cup	2.6

The ideal amount of daily fiber consumption should be **between 30 to 40** grams from fiber rich foods or you can get it with the help of fiber supplements.

What are Antioxidants and Why We Need Them?

The vitamins, nutrients and phytochemicals inside fruits and vegetables are considered **antioxidants**. These powerful substances protect our cells from harm caused by free radicals associated with many types of cancers and heart disease. Free radicals are produced by our natural metabolism but are also stimulated by external factors such as the environment, pollution, contaminated foods, processed foods, etc... **It is essential to consume fruits and vegetables** to fight free radicals and to detox our bodies naturally to live younger and stronger. **Antioxidants diminish the risk of cancer** substantially, eat healthier now and live longer now! Why we need them? Because of their many health powers like **preventing premature aging** and **boosting our immune system** so our bodies are protected against many diseases. But one of the most important reasons why we should take antioxidants is because **they fight free radicals** and detain the early decay of human tissues, organs and cells making us stronger and healthier.

ORAC VALUE
FRUITS

#	Fruit	ORAC
1	Goji Berries	25000
2	Black Raspberries	7750
3	Prunes	5770
4	Bilberry	4460
5	Pomegranates	3300
6	Raisins	2830
7	Blueberries	2400
8	Red Raspberries	2400
9	Blackberries	2036
10	Strawberries	1540
11	Noni Fruit	1505
12	Plums	950
13	Oranges	750
14	Cherries	670
15	Red Grapes	740
16	Red Grapefruit	495
17	White Grape Fruit	460
18	Apples	218
19	Bananas	210
20	Pears	135

WHAT DOES ORAC STANDS FOR?
It stands for Oxigen Radical Absorbance Capacity

WHAT IS THE MEANING OF ORAC?
ORAC IS A WAY TO MEASURE THE ANTIOXIDANT VOLUME IN DIFFERENT FOODS AND SUPPLEMENTS. THE HIGHER THE VALU THE HIGHEST THE VOLUME OF ANTIOXIDANTS THAT FOOD CONTAINS. HIGHER VALUES MEANS HIGHER ANTIOXIDANT POWER TO SLOW DOWN FREE RADICAL DAMAGE AND THE OXIDATIVE PROCESS THAT CAUSES PREMATURE AND THE APPEARANCE OF MANY DISEASES.

EAT MORE FRUITS AND VEGETABLES NOW!

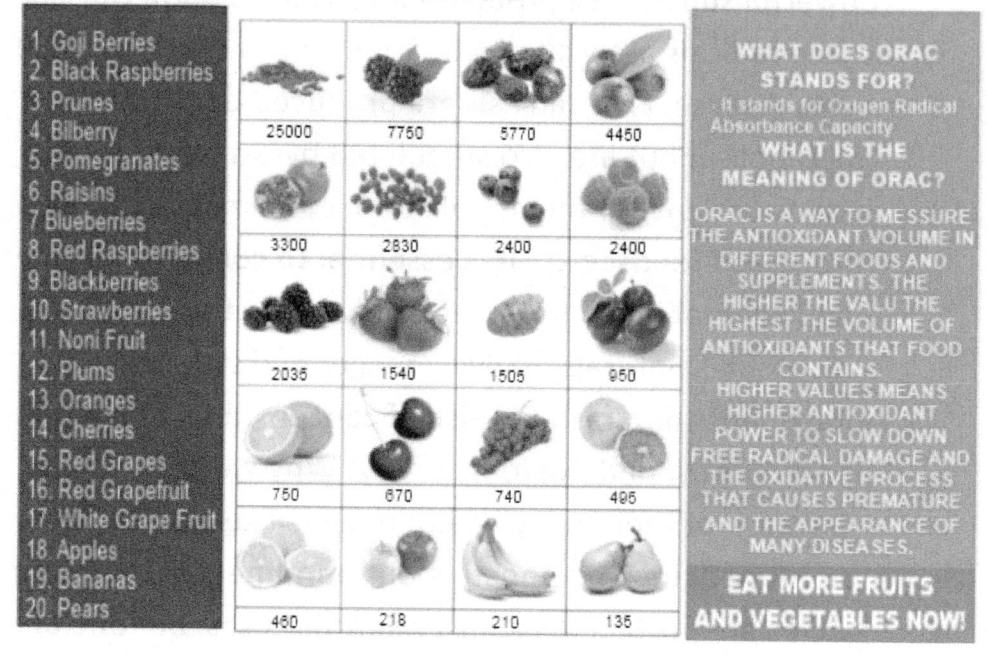

Here is a list of the top vegetables with the most antioxidant powers:

Ginger root, artichokes, lemon balm, garlic, cilantro, coriander, red cabbage, broccoli, red leaf lettuce, asparagus and purple cauliflower.

Being Healthy is Being Happy! – I Wish You a Healthy Life!

Thank you for reading this book and please let me know if you liked it by leaving a positive review

Thank you!

OTHER BOOKS YOU MAY LIKE:

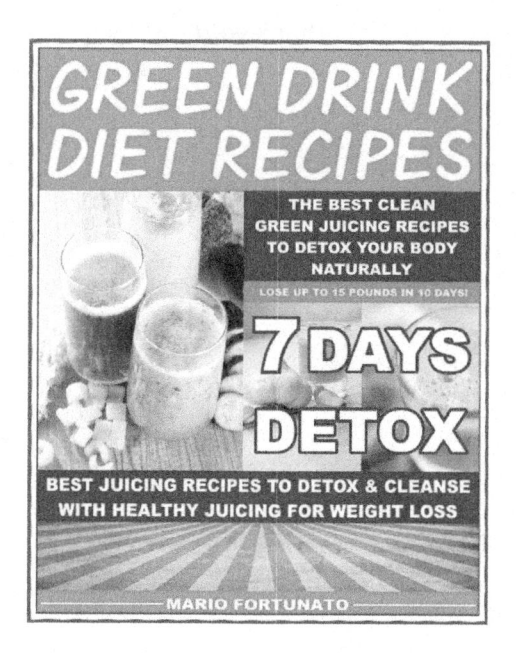

http://tinyurl.com/green-drink-diet

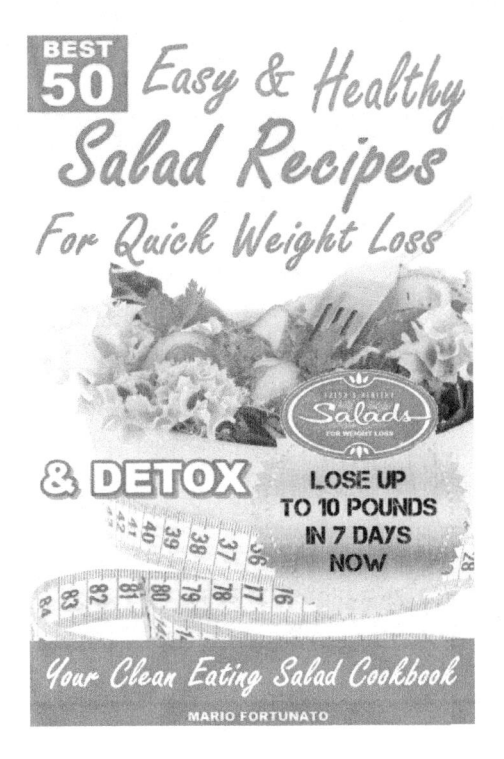

http://tinyurl.com/healthy-salads-book

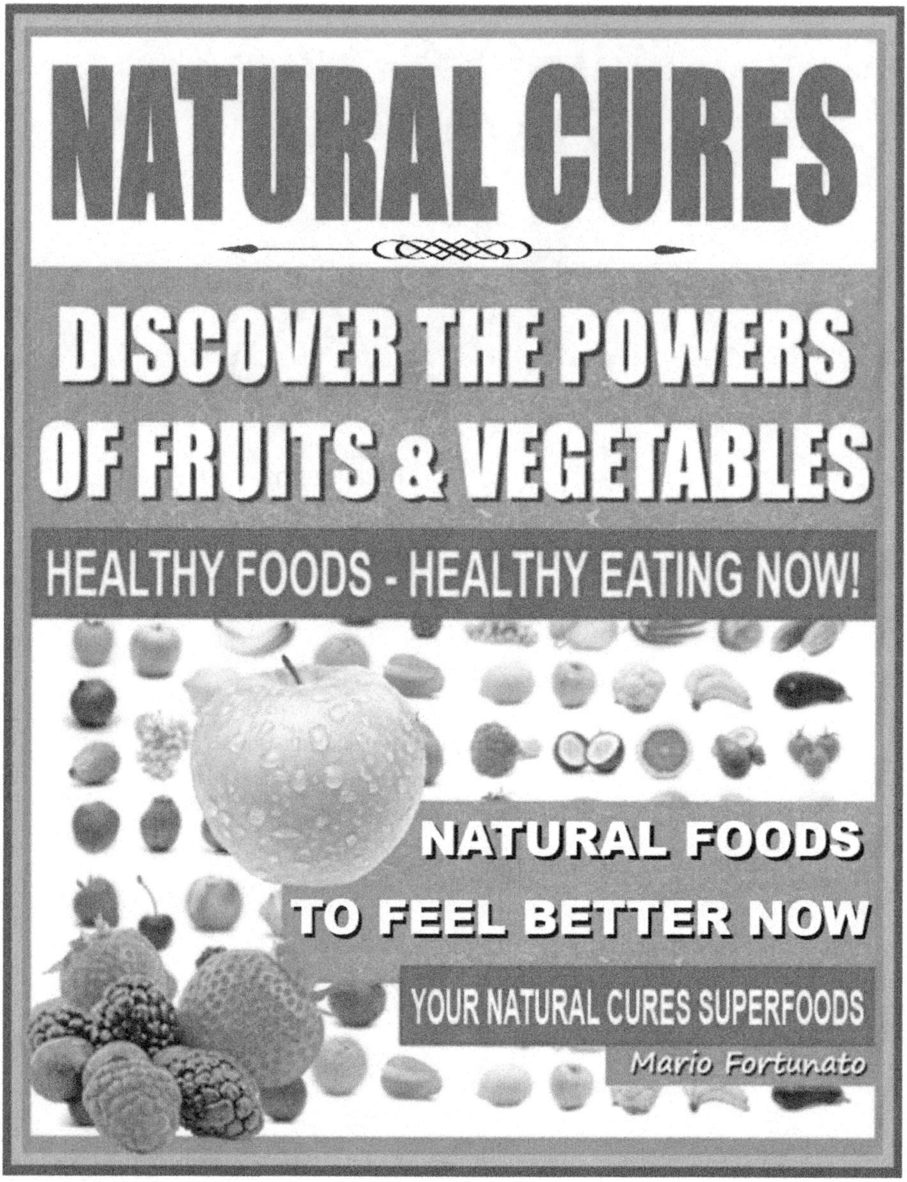
NATURAL CURES
DISCOVER THE POWERS OF FRUITS & VEGETABLES
HEALTHY FOODS - HEALTHY EATING NOW!
NATURAL FOODS TO FEEL BETTER NOW
YOUR NATURAL CURES SUPERFOODS
Mario Fortunato

The information contained in this book is for informational purposes only, and is in no way intended as medical advice or as a substitute for medical counseling. All content and information is provided as-is, and the reader assumes all risks from the use, non-use or misuse of this information. Neither the author or the publisher, partners or affiliates will be held accountable in any way for the use or misuse of the information provided herein. The author and publisher of this work are not medical doctors. This book is not to be considered, in any way medical advice. Because there is some risk involved to make any health changes, all the above mentioned persons involved with the development and distribution of this book are not responsible for any adverse effects or consequences of any kind resulting from the use or misuse of any suggestions or procedures described within this book. Always work with a qualified health professional before making any changes to your diet, prescription drug use, lifestyle or fitness activities.

None of the content should be relied on as a cure, preventive, or treatment for any disease or medical condition. It is recommended that you consult with a licensed medical doctor or physician before acting on any recommendations made in this book.

Health Disclaimer

Any and all information contained herein is not intended to take the place of medical advice from a health care professional. Any action taken based on these contents is at the sole discretion and sole liability of the reader.

Readers should always consult appropriate health professionals on any matter relating to their health and wellbeing before taking any action of any kind concerning health related issues. Any information or opinions provided here are believed to be accurate and sound, however the author assumes no liability for the use or misuse of information provided here.

The author will in any way be held responsible by any reader who fails to consult the appropriate health authorities with respect to their individual health care before acting on or using any information contained herein, and neither the author or publisher of any of this information will be held responsible for errors or omissions, or use or misuse of the information.

Cover apple image courtesy of [MASTER ISOLATED] / FreeDigitalPhotos.net

Cover mixed fruits Image courtesy of [SAILORR] / FreeDigitalPhotos.net

I LOVE YOU

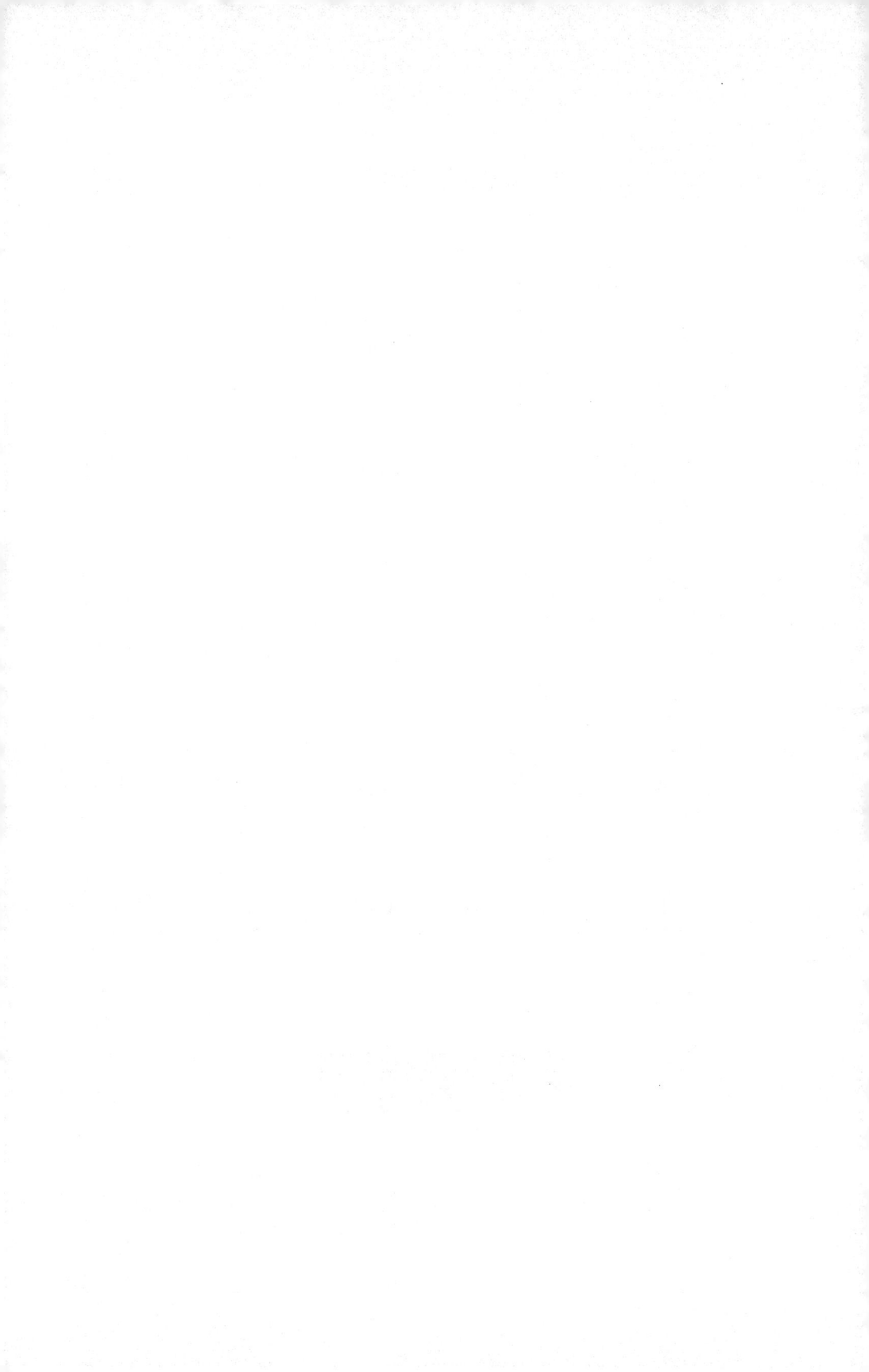

Made in the USA
Middletown, DE
19 April 2024